THE DIGNITY OF THE YOUNG CHILD

How can we keep the young child healthy?
Care and up-bringing in the first three years of life

Michaela Glöckler, Claudia Grah-Wittich (Ed.)

The Dignity of the Young Child

How can we keep the young child healthy?
Care and up-bringing in the first three years of life

Publisher: Verlag am Goetheanum

In coordination with the Association of Waldorf Kindergartens and the
Medical Section at the Goetheanum

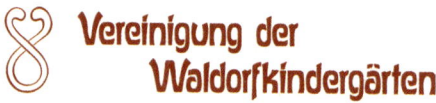

Translated by Astrid Schmitt-Stegmann

www.goetheanum-verlag.ch
Cover design by Wolfram Schildt, Berlin,
usage of photo by Brigitte Huisinga

First edition 2019
© Copyright 2019 by Publisher: Verlag am Goetheanum, CH – 4143 Dornach
All rights reserved
Total production: Gulde-Druck, Tübingen

ISBN 978-3-7235-1615-7

Content

Foreword to the 5th edition *Georg Soldner* 7

Additional Words *Michael Wetenkamp* 9

Foreword to the 4th edition *Michaela Glöckler, Claudia Grah-Wittich* 10

Lectures

Pictures of embryonic development *Michaela Glöckler* 12
How do we promote what only the human being can achieve? *Michaela Glöckler* ... 17
The Dignity of the young child. Ethical motives and challenges *Michaela Glöckler* ... 26
The Dignity of destiny and the arrival on earth *Christoph Meinecke* 40
Autonomy of the young child *Michaela Glöckler* 48
    Examples from the practice *Claudia Grah-Wittich* 55
Concerning the culture of relationships *Michaela Glöckler* 63
    Examples from the practice *Birgit Krohmer* 68
Awakening in the environment *Michaela Glöckler* 73
    Examples from the practice *Claudia Grah-Wittich* 80
An example from the practice *Claudia Grah-Wittich* 86
Educational quality through documentation *Birgit Krohmer* 88

Contributions to the practical work

To receive the child with reverence! *Helmuth von Kügelgen* 99
The pedagogical impulse of Emmi Pikler and Waldorf education *Claudia Grah-Wittich, Brigitte Huisinga* 102
Where do we take children below three? *Brigitte Huisinga* 104
Familiarization in the nursery (crèche) *Ina von Mackensen* 110
The course of the day in the infant care: Wiegestube am «hof» *Brigitte Huisinga* .. 115
To be separate and then together *Claudia Grah-Wittich* 119
The young child is a being of will *Angelika Knabe* 121
The genius of play *Sally Jenkinson* 126
Play-levels *Claudia Grah-Wittich* 131
Caring is education – education is caring *Rolf und Inge Heine* 134
Nutrition for the young child *Petra Kühne* 149
Learning to eat independently in the «Wiegestube» *Brigitte Huisinga* 153
Speech development and speech promotion *Elisabeth Wutte* 157
Speech development through connection *Brigitte Huisinga* 163
Leaving the crèche *Marie-Luise Compani* 165
Working together with parents *Claudia Grah-Wittich* 168

When babies often cry *Ria Blom*	172
Mistreatment and neglect *Madeleen Winkler*	176
The Madonna as source of strength *Hanne Looij*	183

Examples from care facilities

Parent-Child-groups *Brigitte Huisinga*	190

Service – part

Quality indicators for centers catering for the young child	195
Resource addresses	198
Literature	199
About the authors	204
To the pictures	206

Foreword to the 5th edition

This book begins with the development of the unborn and accompanies the paths of the child, his parents, educators, and care takers in the first three years of life in our present time. It conveys a feeling for the dignity of being human, who is in need of connection, care, and warmth from the beginning, and, at the same time, needs to find the way to himself, and learn to express, move and develop himself.

The working together of everyone who accompanies this path from pregnancy, birth and early childhood, as parents, educators, and those in the medical field, is becoming more and more important today. The latest research in pediatrics and education confirm pivotal results of Rudolf Steiner's research that he published already more that a hundred years ago: The first three years are of paramount importance for the child's life-long health, and his capacity to develop (two almost synonymous terms). Parents and educators have the greatest influence at that time and are therefore of central importance. Today's life-style differs fundamentally from the life-style of the previous generations, and the book takes this development fully into consideration. The influence of medicine on the course of pregnancy, birth and early childhood, and also the viewpoint of the parents and educators has increased steadily. Consequently, pediatrics and pedagogy will speak together in this book.

Pregnancy, birth and early childhood is today a topic of focus, a so-called «Care-theme» of the world-wide activity of the Medical Section. It is a part of the School of Spiritual Science founded by Rudolf Steiner, as is the Pedagogical Section. In this field then these two sections are working closely together. «Caring» means nurturing, and this really unites those active in the medical and pedagogical work. Today, the focus is less on the individual, the mother, the pediatrician but rather on the community. No one alone can fully do justice to the child. In the «Care-Group» of the Medical Section, early childhood educators, gynecologists and pediatricians, midwives, nurses, therapists and curative/therapeutic educators work together and try to develop, sustainable, every day concepts on the basis of anthroposophic methodology and general medical and pedagogical research. The purpose is to provide help and orientation for the needs and questions of the many affected in this field. The present book is written by individuals who have cared for the development of the young child for decades.

Parents and educators around the world, are increasingly challenged by the question of how to accompany these first years of the child's life. To accompany these years in such a way that all involved can feel honored in their dignity: The mother who would like to (or must) connect her task as mother and partner (and daughter) with the possibility of professional work beyond the family, as well as being socially active, and to cultivating her own connections. The father who is challenged to recognize his central role to make the most sustainable development possible for the child. Today, he is asked to develop a deeper understanding of the child's early development and needs that go beyond his spontaneous love and joy for playing. This polarity also applies to same-sex parents. The educators are challenged to create a good framework for a group of children of nearly the same age, who draw strongly on the life forces of the adult. The level of stress in general and worldwide has increased due to the many uncertainties during pregnancy and early childhood. This is the case whether we look to the Massai in East Africa or to Baden-Württemberg, as the head of the SPZ at the Olga hospital, Dr. Andreas Oberle reported at the children's health congress in Stuttgart in 2014. We can experience it worldwide. Escape, displacement, traumatic experiences, the fast pace and quick changes of society, the general destabilization in the context of globalization, contribute to the unprecedented change of early childhood.

The present book leads us into the practical. The concepts and key messages of the authors have proven themselves many times in everyday life. Behind these are decades of experience and of development work. The special feature of this work is the close, trusting cooperation of educators and medical professionals who work on a common foundation that focusses on the whole human being. And they consistently check themselves through their practical work in personally founded pedagogical and therapeutic institutions.

It has produced substantial practical knowledge in the field of early childhood education and -care, with a wide dissemination. Therefore, it is hoped that this new and revised edition will also find a wide circulation.

Georg Soldner
Pediatrician,
Deputy of the Medical Section

May 2018

Additional Words

Newborn children touch us, and many people have the immediate impression «they still have a scent of heaven». Caring for children below the age of three is one of those tasks that require the greatest responsibility within a society. Most of what children learn in their life, they already learn before school begins, preeminently in the first three years.

The Association of Waldorf Kindergartens has been working intensively for years in specialty groups on the deepening of pedagogical questions, and on the development of new concepts for the training and further education in the field of early Childhood. At the same time, it is engaged in the founding- and consulting of Waldorf nurseries (crèches).

Several regular early childhood congresses arranged by the Goetheanum in Dornach / Switzerland, as well as specialist conferences give valuable impulses to key questions. It is of great importance to the Association of Waldorf Kindergartens to make this present material available together with the Medical and Pedagogical Sections of the School of Spiritual Science in Dornach, as workbook for teacher training and further education in the field of early childhood as well as for private study. For the 5th edition of this book which has now been published, the articles were reviewed, supplemented, and recomposed.

A special thanks is due to all who prepared, conducted, and documented the Early Childhood Congresses in Dornach.

The present book contains valuable thoughts and descriptions that will be stimulating for the daily work.

Michael Wetenkamp
Executive Member of the
Association of Waldorf Kindergartens

May 2018

Foreword by the editors of the 4th edition

For quite some time the social trend is becoming increasingly prevalent to place the care, nurturing and education of the young child, often just a few months after birth, into the hands of educators and day care mothers, which means, into the hands of professional establishments. The great challenge now is to support parents to remain the primary care givers of their children. For this we must relieve them so that they can move between attachment and freedom. Even if all experts are in agreement that the loving care in the parental home is the «ideal» environment for the young child, the societal development cannot be stopped and demands that the best possible replacement be found.

In view of this development, the young child has increasingly become the focus of general education and also the public. The image of the human being, and the inner attitude in early childhood pedagogy play a central role in this context – also with regard to the question: what keeps the young child healthy?

The significance of the first three years for the individual development of every human being and therefore for their whole biography, shows itself today ever more clearly.

Are the needs and the «dignity of the young child» perceived and respected sufficiently?

It should not be overlooked that irrespective of our behavior as parents or educators, the vitality of the children is increasingly under attack and massively endangered, depending on the cultural area. This is why Waldorf Education attaches great importance to creating opportunities for a healthy and healing development for the very young child. This topic and the questions connected with it were at the center of the third international Early Childhood Congress at the Goetheanum in June 2010. The contributions presented here aim to set a «Milestone» on the topic «The Dignity of the Young Child».

With regard to children under the age of three, we speak less of a «pedagogy for the young child»; rather, it is about the attitude of the adults in their immediate and wider environment. In them, the child orients himself through imitation and carries out the diverse learning processes in a self-active and autonomous way. We need to develop a «situational pedagogy» for the young child which at the same time takes into consideration the global human as well as the local and individual needs of the child – always with the mindset:

What do I model for you?

Such an attitude requires on the one hand a certain selflessness, on the other the ability of conscious self-reflection. The young child – if we consequently think, feel and act out of the understanding of self-development through our destiny – expects from his environment only the inwardly up-right human being as model to imitate. The willingness of the adult to be a role model, and to look inward and learn to work with their own biography knowledgably, and to experience joy in their own change, is the best possible prerequisite for working with the young child. This inward focus that requires consistent practice, turns us into suitable

role models for the constantly practicing child. The Goetheanum as gathering place, above all as «spiritual place», as School of Spiritual Science, is especially suited to develop an attitude of practice. For its inner Foundation Stone was placed with the words:
Practice Spirit-Recalling!
Practice Spirit-Awareness!
Practice Spirit-Beholding!
Upon this is also based the contemplative path for the parents and educators – a path of concentration, of «being in oneself» with the possibility to perceive always new development. This «developmental mood» is the appropriate foundation for the incarnating child.

It is in the nature of anthroposophic medicine and of Waldorf education that they also deal with current research in the medical-pedagogical fields, thereby complementing the results of anthroposophic spiritual research with the natural scientific and practical applications. In addition to the current results concerning brain research, experiences from attachment research, as well as studies from the practical work, e.g. from Emmi Pikler proved especially fruitful.

All contributions work with the process of the incarnating human being in the first three years of life. In order to support the child in his/her development optimally in a world that is often not child-friendly, the interdisciplinary compilation of medical-psychological-pedagogical research approaches has proved to be trend-setting. The first «milestones» of this synopsis are linked to three questions:

How can enough free space be created in the child's environment so that the child can best unfold his innate future capacities? (Movement development, learning to walk)

How can the child's autonomous will to learn be supported and promoted, so that his inner personality can develop on the basis of trust and security? (Speech development, learning to communicate)

How should the environment of the young child be designed, also with regard to the self-education and self-development of the parents and educators, so that the child can experience himself by being by himself but also in connection with his surroundings. (Learning to think)

Dr. med. Michaela Glöckler
Emeritus Leader of the Medical Section of the School of Spiritual Science, Goetheanum (1989–2016)

Claudia Grah-Wittich
Working group of the Young Child in the Association of Waldorf Kindergartens, in Germany

Michaela Glöckler
Pictures of Embryonic Development

I would like to show a few pictures of embryonic development. The schematic presentation[1] shows the first stages of embryonic development.

First Week
In the first week only a sphere is visible, a small cell cluster, the so-called Morula-stage.

Second Week
In the second week a differentiation occurs: One part forms into a delicate spherical sheath, and a second part forms a fine cell line and a small point that expands into a surface, forming a small disc. On one place of this cell circle a densification occurs. We now speak of the germinal bubble. From the small cell cluster, the germinal bubble forms at the beginning of the second week. It looks like a planet in its sphere.

In the following, we will only look at what is formed by this point-shaped cell cluster in the sphere. This is the so-called two-lobed germinal disc which becomes a three-lobed germinal disc: cells migrate from the upper leaf forming a middle cotyledon. The whole thing is disc shaped but it begins the first cleavage stage (Furchenstadium) – it is a wonderful first gesture of uprightness. By the end of the second week the very first conception of the spine is formed, in the design of this line.

Third Week
At the end of the third week, after about 19 or 20 days, a further step of development occurs: The neural tube has already completely folded and the three-foldness into head, middle part and tail is now visible for the first time (Fig.2).

Fourth Week
The following pictures are taken from the atlas of Prof. Blechschmidt from Göttingen[2] who used original embryos which he gently sprayed with wax, to produce original images in magnification.

At the end of the fourth week the size of the embryo is 3,4 mm. We see the head area, the middle area and the tail area (Fig.3). We have to imagine the embryo which now measures about 3 mm as a self-articulated point on the germinal bubble or «sphere» which on closer inspection is extended to be flat and threefold. The leg and arm attachment only appears at the beginning of the second month, in week five.

Fifth Week
The formation of the small arm buds on this threefold human being is among the most touching which can be seen during the embryonic development (Fig. 4).

At this point, the germinal disc begins to transform itself into a sphere – the famous cranial-caudal curvature begins. «Cranio» is the head, and «kauda» is the tail – the head begins to approach the tail.

---

[1] Keith L. Moore, *Embryology*. 3. ed. Stuttgart 1990, p. 34.

[2] Erich Blechschmidt, *Der menschliche Embryo (the human Embryo)*. 2. ed. Stuttgart 1963.

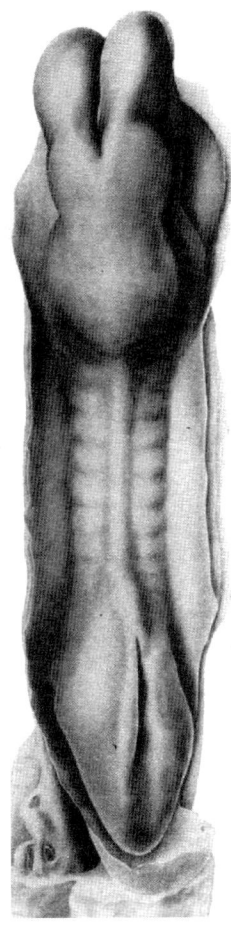

Fig. 2

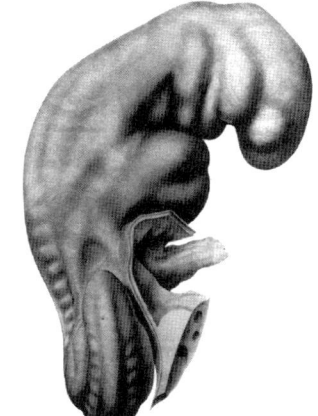

Fig. 3

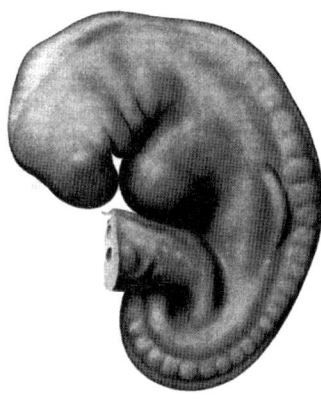

Fig. 4

Rudolf Steiner delineates this development in his lectures «Anthroposophy as Cosmosophy»[3]. He describes how the embryo arranges itself in a circular form, so that the forces from the zodiac can shape or form it equally from all sides. At the beginning of the second months the head and tail have already approached each other, so that the position of the child corresponds to the full zodiac. It thus arranges itself into the cosmos as a whole and no longer behaves as a planet-like point.

This is the moment where the limbs are formed and the will «strikes» into the body. This development continues rapidly. At the end of the fifth week the thick leg bud is already visible. The child is now 6,3 mm tall. (Fig.5, see page 15).

Sixth / Seventh Week

In the middle of the second month the embryo celebrates its one-centimeter-stage, i.e., at the end of the sixth week. Now already the eye system and the otic

[3] Rudolf Steiner, *Anthroposophy as Cosmosophy*. GA 207, GA 208. Lectures of September, October and November 1921.

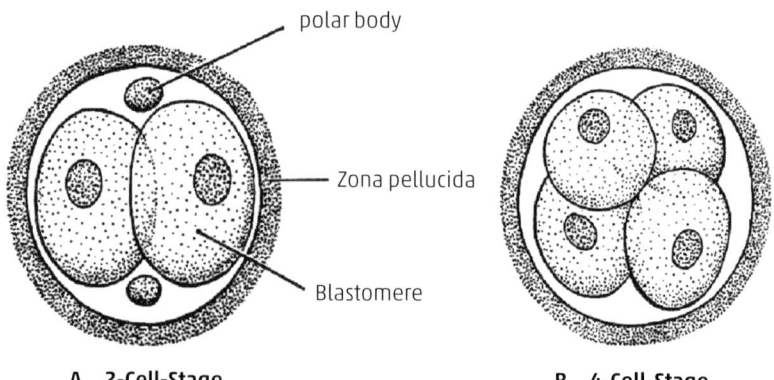

A 2-Cell-Stage **B** 4-Cell-Stage

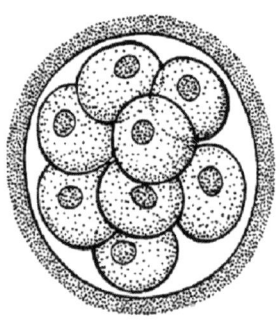

C 8-Cell-Stage **D** Morula

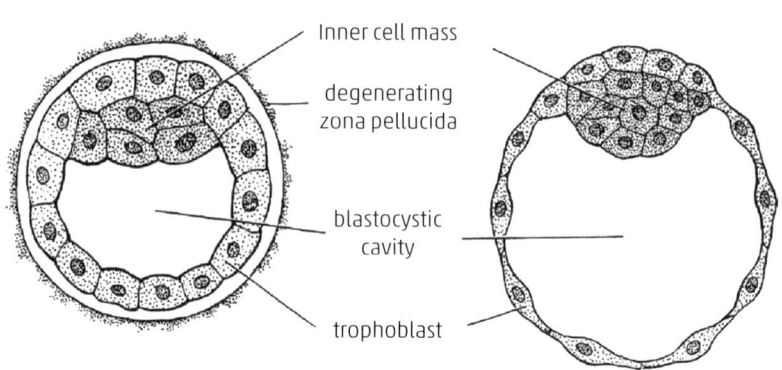

E Early Blastocyst **F** Late Blastocyst

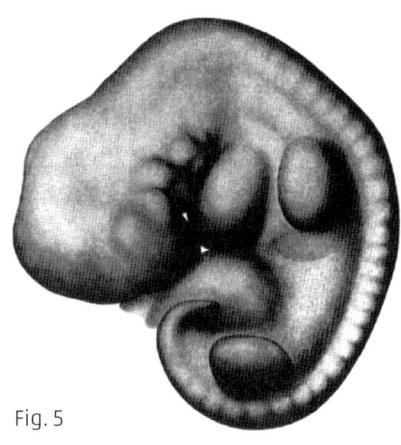

Fig. 5

placode have formed for our most dominant senses. This development correlates with the formation of the fingers and toes. The formation of the peripheral sense organs goes hand in hand with the formation of the «speaking and singing hands». In the beginning you can still see the «webs» between the fingers and toes – the division and differentiation into the separate fingers and toes has not yet taken place. Therefore, we can understand that the use of sleeping pills such as Contergan or alcohol abuse at this age, in the middle of the second month, causes particularly far-reaching and complex damage. In the case of Contergan, there are growth and differentiation inhibitions, especially in the area of the arms so that those affected were born with small fingers on their shoulders because the later onset of growth of the arms was prevented by the drug.

Rudolf Steiner describes in the «Study of Man» how the limbs develop from the periphery: the outermost extension, the fingers and toes come first and that which is closest to the body, the upper arm and thigh, come last. Accordingly, if damage occurs at this early stage, everything that would have grown later, is missing.

Eighth /Ninth Week

At the end of the second month the embryo is 17,5 mm in size which is a good one and a half to two cm tall. The entire organs, including the inner ones, are now created (Fig. 6 and 7, see next page). Therefore, the embryologists state that at this stage the embryonic development is finished. From the third to the ninth month of pregnancy, we speak of the fetal period and of the fetus and not anymore of the embryo. The fetus then continues to grow and thrive and is brought to maturity but the actual shape is completely prefigured after these two months. When a woman normally notices that she is pregnant, all organs are already in place.

In the pictures (Fig. 6 and 7), we can clearly see the large space occupied by the brain and head – practically half of the whole body. From the first structuring the head has the leading position in man; while the limbs attach themselves only later – like appendages – to this giant head, subordinating themselves in the truest sense of the word, to head and trunk.

This short course through the embryonic development, does not only show how complex and «simultaneous» maturation takes place, and how much the human be-

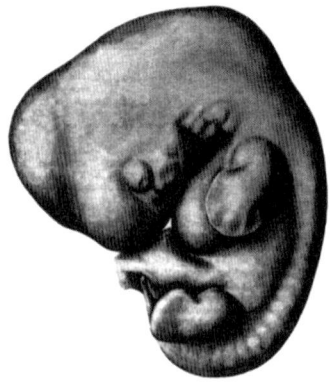

Fig. 6

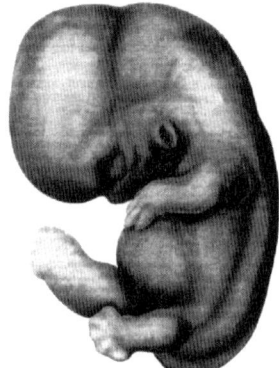

Fig. 7

ing is «human» from the very beginning, it also shows impressively the imagery of evolution itself. Rudolf Steiner's spiritual scientific research and the factual language of the stages of embryonic development show a developmental drama that lets us feel what Friedrich Schiller has his Wallenstein say: *«It is the spirit that builds itself a body.»*[4]

---

[4] Friedrich Schiller (1759–1805), *Wallensteins Tod III*, 13. (Wallenstein's death).

Michaela Glöckler

How do we promote what only the human being can achieve?

Walking – independent acting – shaping of destiny

Walking, speaking and thinking are expression and foundation of our humanity; these abilities are only genetically predisposed as «reaction norms», as we put it in the heredity theory. Depending on the environment and the role model, the child integrates movement patterns and speech sounds.

In connection with walking, speaking, thinking, I would like to focus more closely on the delicate process of the embryonic body building with regard to destiny forming. It can occur that the individuality does not accept the body already formed in the womb of the mother because s/he has the impression that the form of the organs does not fit *that* design that s/he has chosen for their destiny. Then it can come to miscarriages or even after birth to the so-called sudden infant death. On the other hand, we can experience how a child, e.g. of premature birth fights for his life and his body with great strength and is grateful if the intensive medical staff can assist. The acquisition of the upright gait is preceded by intense movement exercises and -procedures of different kinds. For, the embryonic development itself is a constant movement of building and forming. Everything forms itself out of the movement of fluids and movement of cells and cell aggregates. The embryo itself performs wonderful plastic-sculptural, forming and shaping movements. Hands and legs move up and down and splash happily and actively in the amniotic fluid, as long as there is still room.

This forming and shaping movement – in the anthroposophic understanding of man we speak here of the etheric forming forces – is a language of gestures: It is a rounding and stretching, an opening and closing, a penetrating, a coming to rest, and an ending. Growth and development is meaningful movement work.

In the life before birth, spirit and soul exist without the physical body. The communication of the beings in the spiritual world does not happen with word and thought but with a gesture- and sign-language strong in expression, that manifests itself as pure force, pure beingness, pure soul-color, pure form of expression, pure spirit-sound. Translated into earthly concepts, it is a language of manifold gestures and signs, that sounds and sings, has color and form.

In the time before birth, the being of the child, descending through the planetary spheres, enters into dialogue with the hierarchical beings who inhabit these spheres, through gestures and actions. He perceives the indications and signs as challenge how his body should be optimally formed for the next earth life, that it can become a true earthly tool for his future destiny.

Rudolf Steiner describes[1] how the beings in the pre-earthly world are especially interested in everything that happens on the earth. As a thought can move around the whole earthly globe without any trouble, in the same way are these pre-earthly

---

1 Rudolf Steiner, *Life between Death and Rebirth*. GA 140, Anthroposophic Press 1968, lecture 11. Oct. 1913, p. 353 ff.

beings still totally without space or time. They are omnipresent through their consciousness. Corresponding with their destiny they are now beginning to choose, to group themselves, and perhaps become inspired by one human being, a poet or a scientist who lived on earth a hundred years before they themselves are born. Rudolf Steiner mentioned that those as yet unborn live in future oriented human motives and through this they gain courage and inspiration for the new earth life.

Later, when they have decided where they want to go a tragic battle often ensues. They recognize that they need a certain bodily disposition. It can often happen – according to Rudolf Steiner – that parents who can offer a suitable germinal system and/or live at a place, where one would like to meet an important human being, are psychologically and morally not easy so that childhood or youth will be difficult. The alternative would be, to find a loving environment for childhood and youth but to forego meeting important individuals. This discrepancy that happens before the embryonic development, many of the unborn souls would experience as a painful battle. However, this also sheds a light onto the realm of freedom on the earth: On the one hand there shine forth inspiring role models from this earth across to the world of the stars, on the other hand the infinitely tragic experience of the indicated battle.

In the beginning young children take up what humans do in the same way that they had taken up the activity of the angels and archangels, they imitate it. It is against this background that we can understand why they do not only imitate the outer gestures but – as they were accustomed to in the spiritual world – also the moral gestures and the movements of thoughts and feelings of human beings. The period of imitation is a gradually fading process of the behavior patterns from the pre-earthly world. Only after that do children begin to place themselves more and more on their own feet, first bodily, then soul-spiritually, and then learn to determine their actions themselves.

Our topic is called: How do we promote what only the human being can achieve?

How then, do we best support learning to walk?

The child first perceives the impulse for uprightness of the body with the tentative gaze of the eye. From the first lifting of the head shortly after birth, he has the striving for uprightness when lying on the stomach. However, he must first prepare his body for the upright standing – therefore walking begins with learning to stand. Therefore, a decisive stage between lying down and learning to walk is an extended crawl phase; because in the four-footed walking (vierfuesslergang) during the crawl-phase the spine is in the best relaxed position and mobile, so that he can adapt well to the weight load when standing upright. The next step is that children pull themselves up on a chair or a low table. Crawling and pulling-up must alternate as much as possible in this first period, so that the back muscles become strong enough to sustain the constant balancing while standing.

When standing and walking all muscles are involved, not only the legs. We should know that. Therefore, standing and learning to walk really means raising the whole human being into the vertical but in such a way, that it swings elastically. We human beings always are in a fragile balance; we are not stable like an animal on its four legs. In order to keep our balance, we must always raise ourselves actively into the vertical. This does not happen by itself. We can tell by the fact that drunks or very tired people fall more easily – and forward. When standing, we have to practice «restraint» in the truest sense of the word because our natural focus is somewhat forward.

This restraint is not only a body-language-gesture but an eminently important moral force. The human being who knows no restraint, «does not stand on his own feet». He is more often exposed to his own emotions than a person who stands upright or in restraint. When we as adults practice to balance the I in the feeling between the thinking and willing pole, we can directly feel it.

One more thought about freedom: Every joint, knee-joint, wrist-joint etc. has gradations of freedom. We usually move out of a spontaneous need to move somewhere, to reach for something. Nowhere is freedom so directly experienced as in movement. Giving space and freely letting the urge to move manifest is the most important remedial measure, in order to let a child experience freedom. In this context it is important to form the course of the day and the environment so that you interfere as little as possible with the spontaneous movements and activities of the children. Learning to walk and move should be connected with a basic experience of freedom.

When the human being has learned to walk, then he is also able to walk towards others. With this the precondition is created to accept destiny, to walk towards one's destiny. When we walk towards something, we shape relationships in space through our movement. Through the uprightness, we create a relationship between below and above, between right and left, between in front and behind. Towards the back, towards the past, we seem closed. To the front we are open – we orient ourselves to the future, where something will continue. We show the past that we are finished with it, and we move into the future.

Learning to walk also signifies, forming a meaningful relationship to space and to develop this further. That is why it is so important, that the objects in a room are placed in a meaningful order, and that the people interact with each other in a mindful way.

Speaking – Listening – Ability to Love
Speaking begins with listening. The larynx must first develop itself into a speaking tool. In the infant it is still located a little bit too high and that for a good reason: This allows the infant to drink and breathe at the same time. On the epiglottis and on the mucosa of the trachea there are still taste buds, which later regress. During the first year, the larynx slowly descends. Then the children stop breathing when they swallow.

In mammals, the larynx remains in this «baby-position» all their life. That is why they can only make inarticulate sounds and screams. Nor can the animals train their lips, teeth, and palate for speaking because the larynx remains in that position and the palate does not curve. The larynx never becomes an instrument for speech. Therefore only the forming of certain sounds is possible – depending on the formation of the mouth- and palate curve.

I would now like to give some practical indications for remedial measures with regard to learning to speak.

How can speech be promoted by a good role model?

At this point I would like to emphasize the importance of non-verbal speech. Speech development with the young child, especially in the first three years, is best done through «speaking actions», where children can experience that everything that is done has meaning. Watching is like listening at this age. The experience of the meaningful is the incentive either to do it also or to say something meaningful. Today we talk far too much at children and explain too much – and very little of this talk is an expression of deeds and has weight.

The most important elements of speech development are meaningful, expressive, skillful movements and words, that correspond with deeds. Children can distinguish very well whether words have weight or not. If not, they do not take them seriously. Then they provoke on and on, until the adult is absolutely furious and gives up, just lets them go ahead. That, however is a disappointing experience, because they do not have the example of an adult who stays with what he said.

It is important that we ourselves articulate well. 60 to 70 percent of the Kindergarten children have speech problems today. This is a consequence of lack of articulation when we speak to the children.

We need all our muscles not only for standing and walking but also for speaking. In order to articulate well we need all muscles. For, when we speak our larynx with its small support- and muscle apparatus executes all movement in miniature that we make with our fingertips, hands, arms and legs when we move them. That is why the healthy development of movement is such an essential precondition for learning to speak.

A further aspect is the speech melody. In it lives the feeling element of the language. Its carrier is the vowel. Vowels are music. They give the very individual sound to the speech. The consonants form and end this sound stream. We are always forming sound streams and ending them – this is what we call speaking.

This simple observation shows that two aspects are very closely connected in speech:
- One aspect is what the human being experiences in his soul and wants to make known through sound as a mood, as a statement, to the outside – via the vowels.
- The other is that which forms the speech stream with the help of the speech tools, musculature, teeth and palate –

the consonants, they interrupt the stream, hold it back, squeezing it.

It is something inward and something outward, an air stream and the speech tools – that we connect when we speak, a communion, that happens within ourselves. Speech always shapes what the human being wants to experience and communicate in and around the world and with others.

When speaking, we form and shape relationships in time, in the here and now. Listening too occurs in time. We can also say that speech occurs in time and simultaneously shapes time, transcending relationships. For, I can talk about the past and bring it into the present. But I can also plan the future and start with it now. The present mediates between both – it is the space where we speak. This explains why the Archangel Michael is only interested in the future. Rudolf Steiner put it this way in his notebook: «*Michael does not live with the causes but with the consequences of human deeds.*»[2] In face of a problem it is only important to ask oneself:

What can I learn from this?
How has this problem changed me?
How do I use this pain that woke me up, in order to do something meaningful for the future?

That is Michaelic thinking, that communicates itself by speech. With one word, we can finish the past and can decide to forgive or to ask for forgiveness, and begin anew.

Which spirits do we ask to be our guests when we speak?

- Christ says: «*Where two or three come together in my name, there I will be among them.*»[3]
- Lucifer says: Where two insist on their standpoint in my name, there I am in the midst of them.
- Ahriman says: Where two are fighting with each other in my name, there I am in the midst of them.

In the way we speak with each other, we call very different qualities of beings and qualities of working into our inter-human relationships. The spirits that we call by their name through our behavior, are truly present whether we like it or not.

It had always been a concern of my father[4] to emphasize that the spiritual world is not in the hereafter, but in the here and now. And just as Christ has his messengers and helpers in all hierarchies, Lucifer and Ahriman also have certain fallen angels as their servants and helpers.

In the lectures that Rudolf Steiner gave in Prague in 1923[5], he states that it is the task of the educator to prepare the children through speech for the experience of the night, so that they can bring back strengthening forces from the realms of the Christ-connected angelic beings and not demonic inspirations.

---

2 Rudolf Steiner, *World History in the Light of Anthroposophy*, GA 233, Rudolf Steiner Press, 1977.
3 Matthäus Kap. 18, Vers 20. (Gospel of St. Matthew)
4 Dr. Helmuth von Kügelgen – *14. Dezember 1916 † 25. Februar 1998.
5 Rudolf Steiner, *The Human Soul and its connection with Divine-Spiritual Individualities*, GA 224, Lectures of 28. and 29. April 1923.

Thinking – Self-awareness – Spirit-knowledge

In a verse for Pentecost by Rudolf Steiner[6] we read:

*Creature ranks
with creature in the width of Space,
Creature follows creature in the
rounds of Time.
Linger, oh Man, in widths of Space,
in rounds of Time
Yet mightily your soul rises above them
When you divine or knowingly
behold the Eternal
Beyond the confine of Space,
beyond the flow of Time.*

The ability to think reaches beyond spatial limits and conditions of time. This capacity lives in the first years as unconscious intelligence in the child. Then – often suddenly, as with a jolt – the child gains the consciousness: I am an I. Often scary experiences provoke this, but sometimes also happy feelings or an especially peaceful experience, where the child for the first time awakens to himself as thinking being. In thinking every human being leads his/her very own, very personal, «supersensible» life that begins with the first fully conscious announcement of «I». It is important that as educator we develop a warm understanding for this third decisive step in early childhood development: The awakening to oneself. The philosopher Fichte liked to do the following thought exercise with his students: «*Gentlemen, please look at this wall – and now, gentlemen, think this wall, imagine this wall with closed eyes vividly. And now, dear gentlemen, think the one who thought the wall*».

This thought exercise makes us realize that we are also someone in thinking, a pure «thought», willed, formative, active potential – a thought-being-, not only a body-being. The more references we create between us and the world when we think, the less isolated we view things, the more we integrate them into the overall context, the more truthful is what we think. We use thinking to learn everything that we as human beings cannot do naturally – that is, instinctively – e.g.

- in order to get a reasonable structure into the course of our day,
- in order to learn to sleep in the right way,
- in order to learn to eat right,
- in order to become socially competent,
- in order to pursue self-, human- and world knowledge,
- in order to reproduce ourselves in a dignified way,
- in order to be employed and to be able to cope with life – etc.

With all this, we need to engage our consciousness, recognize mistakes, undergo learning processes. Animals naturally have what we must wrestle to achieve. With them learning is all about the body instincts. They have no other choice but to behave intelligently. But they are not capable of unfolding free will nor are they capable of life-long learning and change.

In the case of mineral, plant and animal, knowledge, the law of nature, the underlying wisdom of development, is bound

---

[6] Rudolf Steiner, *The Reappearance of Christ in the Etheric*. GA 118, lecture, 15. Mai 1910.

to substance, to the genetic material. Nowhere does this wisdom, the lawfulness according to which everything functions, appear «by itself», detached, independent of matter. It is always tied to a real process.

Human thinking is the only place where the laws of nature can be found in abstract form, extracted from matter. The wisdom of the world emerges there from the natural existence and leads in our consciousness a separate spiritual existence. That is why we experience our thinking as light and free, without weight, not binding. Thinking is pure spirit movement, without realizing anything materially. We can think everything that exists and find all laws that are followed by creation and the evolution of the world – a pure spirit play, lifted out of the natural earthly evolution of the world.

We may reflect on the thoughts that the Creator God has realized. But not only that. Even plants and animals «think» the creation by living it and materially embodying this wisdom. We humans can turn thinking into a creative process, into thinking of things that have not yet existed, and can thereby change the world and life.

But we can also think nonsense and error in a completely free play of possibilities. We shape our reality according to our thinking: hands and feet have to wait till we tell them what to do, where they should go. They are subordinate to thought as we can see from the upright human posture[7].

---

[7] Rudolf Steiner, *The Human Soul and its connection with Divine-Spiritual Individualities*. GA 224, *Drei Etappen des Erwachens der menschlichen Seele*. Lecture of 28. April 1923.

In this respect today, we face the shocking fact that the creation from the origin has reached a critical phase. It is up to us, to our free decision how it will continue with us and with the world.

The gods have called man the «crown of creation», they have not physically completed him, have not created him to be as perfect as the animals. We were created as half physical and half spiritual beings but not in such a way that we can find in the cradle the «how to use» instructions, how the infant should use his spirit in life, but in such a way that he has to find this himself.

Just as man must hold himself back a bit when he achieves uprightness, in order to hold himself in balance and to move freely to all sides, so too has the Logos, the Creator God held back in man: He gave us what was left over from the original creative process as personal creative power. He has refrained from perfecting the human and with this gesture gave us the freedom to use this innate creative power the way we wish. We have this latitude of freedom in our thinking, there we are absolutely free, thanks to the restraint of God. We unfold our self confidence in the world of thought that gives us all the laws, all the creative possibilities, but does not determine us. Therefore, the intelligence can also be at the service of lies, and destructive activity, as in crime and war.

I would like to take a further step in this spiritual reality and show how the human being does not lose himself in all this spirituality but find himself. For, thinking does not overpower us but makes it possible to have a conscious relationship with the spirit.

Scotus Eriugena, a theologian and monk of the early Middle Ages, said in his book De *Devisione naturae* (About the Division of Nature) that the human being shares the physical substance with the minerals, life with the plants, the soul with the animals, and with the angels thinking. However, he asks:

> What does the human being only have for himself? Where is he all alone, totally self-sufficient, and can thank himself for what he does?

His answer is that only the human being has the capacity to judge. When he judges, he is totally placed on himself. When judging, he tries to see the parts in a coherent relationship with the whole and to see in this way the truth of a situation or a process. We human beings are the «beings of judgment», as it is stated in the Old Testament, and should be able to decide between good and evil. Self knowledge and self assessment, world knowledge and world assessment is added by the human being as new quality to the given creation. Rudolf Steiner takes the comparative observation of Scotus Eriugena further in his work. He shows what we owe to the hierarchies and the Holy Trinity, and how the whole creation process looks from the view point of the spirit:

- We owe thinking to the Angels.
- Feeling, together with our ability to express ourselves and have speech, we owe to the Archangels, other places also called «Spirits of Language».
- We owe our will to the Archai, the «spirits of time», so that we can create something in time for the development of ourselves and the world.
- We can thank the Exusiai, the «Spirits of Form», that we can experience ourselves as individual being, as «I», that can relate to everything and can judge spiritually.
- The Dynamis, the «Spirits of Movement», we can thank that we can move and change.
- The Kyriotetes, the «Spirits of Wisdom», we can give thanks to them for our ability to experience wisdom filled connections. Anthroposophy, the «Wisdom of Man», is a gift of these Kyriotetes.
- To the Thrones, the «Spirits of Will», we owe the will to become human: the wish to learn, the drive to learn, the will to develop.
- To the Cherubim, the «Spirits of Harmony», we owe our conscience that strives to bring all that is problematic into balance again, to bring peace even if this is at times not possible until a future life.
- To the Seraphim, the «Spirits of Love», we give thanks that the whole creation is penetrated by love, and that we have a personal destiny that never leaves us – that surrounds us as possibility to learn to make the best of all that happens to us, and never to despair. This highest hierarchy stands directly before the countenance of God.

Now a look at the Holy Trinity, the Father, the Son, the Spirit:

1. Everything that underlies creation and our existence in connection with the

world is grounded in the Father God. The Father God wishes that we should be joyful. The virtue that furthers learning to walk and furthers movement development, is joy, the joy of movement.
2. From the principle of the Son emanates the possibility of the continued development of the world. The Son wishes that we are honest when we speak, leaving others free, and that we treat each other in a loving way. Decisive is the will for truth and honesty, for without truth freedom and love are not of much value.
3. To the principle of the Spirit we owe the possibility to take our own development individually and independently into our hand. In thinking we are spiritually at home: It carries us from the time before birth through earthly life into the after death experience. It is the indestructible etheric world in which we may trust. We experience our will in thinking as something that has being, that establishes our spiritual existence and is capable of helping us and healing us and others.

Michaela Glöckler
The Dignity of the Young Child – Ethical Motives and Challenges

About the global mission of infant care (day nurseries / crèches)

Children are born into a great variety of cultural conditions around the world: The Middle-European situation is completely different from that in South America or that in the Eastern countries. All the more surprising, therefore, is the extent to which infants are international beings. They are still completely open to cultural and social imprints. If I bring an infant from Japan to Switzerland, s/he will soon speak Swiss-German and adjust totally to the local conditions. And when I do the opposite, I take a Swiss infant from Emmental to Tokyo, he will speak Japanese. There is no other way. Today's brain researchers say the brain of the infant is plastic and impressionable. But this applies to the whole body of the infant, or toddler.

A cultural change for humanity has greater chances when we have an eye on this universal aspect of early childhood in our care facilities. Nurseries are the ideal starting point for the development of more humanity across the earth – I say this very consciously –, because the parents bring their children out of their own free will, release them, so to speak, out of the close ties with culture- and family into a free space of education.

Each one of us has his own concerns: lack of money, low pay, insufficient space, difficult, frustrated parents, colleagues who are ill or with whom we cannot work well together. Perhaps we can look beyond these regional issues and ask, how we ourselves can begin to build a global network of a genuinely international education towards human dignity. The faster we develop brotherhood in the service of our children the better it is for them. Before God and the young child with his/her infinite willingness to develop, and their joy in it, we are all equal. We adults who have perhaps already given up a little on development could learn a lot from children in this regard. For in a climate in which children's joy of development can live, the best inspirations will come to us.

The deeper meaning of infant care in a nursery/crèche environment

The meaning of nursery education cannot only be to keep children as well as possible so that nothing will happen to them, and they get what they need until they are handed back again to the parents. To support them in their development, to give the human being space to help develop spirit, soul and body should always be the ultimate goal.

It also means, that we as care givers strive to experience in all the details of daily life the inner truth of the outer material processes.

If you, for instance, turn on the light somewhere, we can explain this shining light totally materialistically as an electromagnetic phenomenon.

But how do I experience the light as human being?
What is the being of light?

When it lights up, things immediately appear in context. When I close my eyes, it becomes inwardly light, because my thinking has light structure. A thought is light;

when we understand something, it lights up in us. When I look at something with loving interest in day light, I experience the divine aspect of my soul – then my humanity shines forth, the higher part in me. Inner and outer light come together.

Please, do not believe that it is one and the same for the young children that you care for the understanding you have of light, when you turn on the light in the morning; whether you think of nothing or of electrons and electric wiring or whether you know what you do soul-spiritually and bodily when you turn on the light in a room. Only when you also turn on the light inwardly, the moment you turn it on outwardly are you truly human. Whether we really educate for truth, beauty and goodness depends also on this, that we have interest to find out, e.g., the truth of the light.

What is the Truth of Water?

We should pose this question to ourselves when we bathe a child. Externally, water is an interesting chemical substance that has the ability to absorb, dissolve and mediate between all water soluble substances.

But what is water seen in a soulful, moral way?
Why does it say in the gospel that the water moved by an angel takes in healing forces?
What does water have to do with angels?

Once you bring together all you know about water then you will see: It is the epitome of «service». The moral quality of being available wherever and whenever one is needed. In this all-embracing form, only the water has this total availability. It is therefore, the epitome of selflessness, and we can understand that angels have a lot to do with water. Angels are like water: They accompany us through births and deaths, are always selflessly available but do not interfere with our freedom. However, they are – just like the water itself – completely themselves. The human being can only become «self-less» when he has become inwardly strong enough that he can «let go» of himself without fearing to lose himself. Rudolf Steiner remarked: «*Only the self-reliant man can be available*».

When we become conscious of what we are doing when washing an infant or toddler, when we are true and honest and let the truth of the water live in us, then we wash the child in angel-substance. Then s/he can physically experience what the Guardian angel is spiritually: purity, gentleness, transparency, clarity, cleanliness, morality, regeneration, healing, comfort, refreshment.

Love as Cultural Task

The leading picture of the work in infant care seems extraordinarily demanding and hard to fulfill. An infant care educator or a young mother can easily get the feeling that they cannot meet this high standard. There is, however, one capacity that can compensate for all inability – love.

What can help us to master the challenges of educating despite our own inability?

Nature has arranged it so that a mother instinctively loves her child. Since God knew, how difficult everything else is, he gave to love a wonderful natural side, that is in our blood and makes us attractive to one another, even if we are not very developed and immoral. This kind of love works already when we only see the baby. We must be very hardened if we do not at least smile a little when we see a baby. We have a natural love for young children. On this natural love that is very individual, we can rely to a certain degree. When *this* love fails, our human instincts fail. Then we are already on the verge of needing therapy.

This natural capacity for love must be further developed to become a love capacity of the soul that is independent from its natural foundation. If I wish to raise a child of someone else, I need this soul culture.

- On the spiritual level, love is identical with truth and wisdom. Here we speak of an understanding with the heart.
- On the soul level love can become master over our antipathies and sympathies; love conquers envy, jealousy, and hate, but also fanatic sympathy. It releases one-sided emotions, harmonizes them and creates honest, objective human relationships.
- On the physical level it expresses itself as instinct, drive, inclination and feeling and gives us direct access to one another independent of the degree of progress of our soul-spiritual development.

Involving the Parents

When we speak about care for the infant in the first three years of life, we may not even think of the children without their parents. It would already be an insult if we would lose the parents out of our consciousness, as soon as they delivered the children at the door. Then we would not do justice to the children nor the parents.

At this early age it is about a very different kind of up-bringing than later, when the children are older. In the first years of life the child is completely open to his environment; s/he experiences herself as part of the whole. The more we carry this whole in our consciousness as care taker, the more comfortable the child feels.

It is important to raise a picture in one's mind in the evening of the people who are most closely connected with this child: the grandmother or other people that deliver the child in place of the parents. It takes practice, until you succeed to bring into an inner picture the child and what you have learned about his home. Of course, you cannot go through every parent's house in detail when you come home at night exhausted. This is not what is meant. When you do something with the child, you should see first and foremost a picture of the mother before you, when she showed herself most clearly as herself. This enhances the experience of security and of wholeness in the child. We have to envisage the whole thing – albeit discretely and inwardly.

Motherhood and Occupation
Is motherhood a natural task or an occupation?

This is a wonderful topic to argue about. I myself am of the opinion that motherhood is both. It is a profession which means that there are also mothers for whom this is not the right profession, they wish for something different. For my mother it was *the* occupation, and I am still today deeply grateful to her. But my mother also had to sacrifice a great deal, and she was not always at one with her fate as a graduated chemist, environmental advocate, and educator, not to be able to enter fully into a professional life because of her six children. We children also noticed that now and then. Therefore, certain questions formed in me early, e.g. whether one can say in principle that it is best for children when mother is at home, and the mother should «actually» only think of herself when the children are out of the house. We do not help the children nor our contemporaries when we hang on to principles. The age of principles expires the moment individual freedom begins and with it individual responsibility.

So why are principles no longer up-to-date?

Because they lead to immaturity. If I have principles, I know from the beginning what is right and what is wrong. Then I do not even have to check or consider whether the principle is also valid in the current situation or whether an exception should be made and, whether under these circumstances something completely different would be due. According to such a principle, the mother should be with her children in the house in the first three years. This principle is indeed right for the child and the best, but it does not meet the reality of life. And when I follow the principle with clenched teeth, I'm far from being a good mother. Conversely, a mother giving her child to a day mother or a nursery is far from being a bad mother – on the contrary. If she looks forward to seeing her child in the afternoon or evening and picks him/her up from a good day care or nursery without a guilty conscience, everyone is served. The childcare center has a professional work place, the mother her professional job, and the baby or little child is well cared for.

In the pediatric office hours, I often dealt with mothers who were highly idealistic and wanted to «do everything right», but were not really coping with their destiny of having a child. These mothers were suffering pangs of conscience and feelings of guilt, to the point of depression because they wanted a different life- and work perspective for themselves. They certainly had wished for a child at some point – but not right now!

The «as-well-as» of the anthroposophic life practice

Here is a wonderful feature of Anthroposophy: on the one hand, it can be said from Anthroposophy that it would be ideal for the child if he could stay at home with his mother during the first three years because he feels best there. On the other hand, you can give deep comfort to desperate mothers, and convey to them that it is more important for the child, to have a content, happy, engaged, although perhaps a little stressed mother in the morning and in the evening, on weekends and during the holidays, but a mother who can identify both with herself and with life, than to be spending the whole day as a housewife wanting to make everything perfect, but struggling with herself and her destiny. For, if there is no happy, loving, life affirming atmosphere at home where the child is often smiled at, then it is much better that the child spends the day in a nursery where he is motivated and professionally cared for.

The more individual and optimal Anthroposophy is translated into the practical life as a family culture, the better it is for family and day care nursery. It would be wonderful if we could add a parent school where mothers who are interested in motherhood as profession would have the opportunity to learn this profession. Mothers who have opted for a different profession should be able to pursue it with clear conscience because they bring their child to us into the nursery, and we enjoy our work. As far as the weekend is concerned, we should ask the parents to keep some of the good ideas and habits, so that the child has some continuity and security, even on days when s/he is not in the nursery. We give them as much as they can implement – not too much and not too little and as tactful, but also as honestly as possible.

This is how, the «as-well-as», this golden rule of the consciousness soul, could look in concrete situations. If we follow this rule as much as possible, we will do justice to our lives, our children, our parents, but also to our self-education.

I would like to pursue the question of the self-confidence that parents and educators need to meet the demands.

Working on a healthy Self-awareness

To have self-awareness means that we know about ourselves. Today everyone works more or less strongly on his «outfit». This self-confidence propped up by the outside is, however, very vulnerable as is the one that supports itself with the so-called latest state of science. I will only name the magic word «Brain-Research». When something is «proven» by brain research, it is immediately cited and translated into educational maxims. The «knower» thus feels strengthened in his self-confidence.

In what ways have we perhaps become dependent – on the knowledge of others?

Who really is pondering and asking himself whether the new educational maxims really make sense?

But there are two further levels of self-awareness through self-discovery which we not only have to develop within ourselves but above all, we should lay the groundwork for this in young children: self-experience on the soul level and self-experience on the spiritual level through thinking.

How can we come to Self-experience on the Spiritual level?

People who were imprisoned or tortured describe what kept them alive and helped them to overcome their traumatization: They had certain thoughts, images, people, that seemed to them very vivid as if present – this could also be those who have died or supersensible beings who suddenly came as mental representations to give comfort. When we become self-aware in this indestructible realm of thought then we experience ourselves as spiritual beings among spiritual beings. Then our self-awareness stabilizes «from inside» and is not dependent anymore on outer recognition. We can visualize our spiritual being only in that part of the human being that is as eternal and indestructible as a thought. And we can keep the relationship with the deceased only in thoughts and feelings, those pure soul-spiritual abilities, and can see in images before us, what physically does not exist.

In thoughts and feelings, the spiritual world can reveal itself: The good spiritual beings can embody themselves in good thoughts and feelings, while our hateful, ugly thoughts attract devilish and demonic beings that attack us with fear, pangs of conscience and feelings of guilt. We have to discover that we are spiritual and therefore thought-penetrated beings but that we are also soulful and therefore feeling-penetrated beings.

It is one of Rudolf Steiner's most far-reaching research outcomes to have discovered the identity of life- and thought forces (he calls them etheric forces, and the sum of life activity, and regeneration forces, ether body/etheric organism) and to have made them fruitful for pedagogical and medical practical work. Our thought life that we experience as our spiritual inner life is our body free potential, which is not used anymore for the growth of the body.[1]

---

1 Rudolf Steiner, Ita Wegman, *Grundlegendes für eine Erweiterung der Heilkunst nach geisteswissenschaftlichen Erkenntnissen*. GA 27, 1. Kapitel.

Adults who are aware that the human being establishes his self-awareness on the spiritual level, in the eternal, through thinking and that this will be retained for them in the spiritual world after death, create thoughts and feelings in which something indestructible lights up. These thoughts and feelings create an atmosphere that allows the infants and toddlers to take them up as qualities from the environment through imitation and use these to build up their physical body.

Sensory care and Self-consciousness

The most important thing is this: When I learn to think in this way, I also know what I need to do with the children in my care. Then I understand, why there is nothing more important in the first years of life, especially in the first year, then the care of the senses.

For, with every sense experience self-experience is made possible. A child cannot yet experience herself on the thought level, only the adult can do that. S/he can only experience herself through sense experiences. The meaning of all development is to work to acquire a soul-spiritual presence and for the outer world a suitable self-awareness.

When we devote all of our energy to help children in the first and second year of life gain a healthy self-awareness, we save them much work and effort later on.

They can then have their entire will available to work for their fellow human beings and contribute to find solutions for problems.

With the sense of balance we grasp the whole human being; it brings about the integration of the movement possibilities. The sense of touch on the other hand, is the key sense for self-perception, from outside via surface sensibility and from inside via depth sensibility. I only experience myself in my earthly body when I bump into something. The depth sensibility is so important because it allows the organs of our body to perceive each other and to coordinate with each other. The surface sensibility gives us the consciousness of enclosure, of unity of the self in relation to the multiplicity of the organs and functions.

We can see then that health and illness but also the quality of self-experience depend on the key senses. However, they are only the representatives for all the other senses. When all twelve senses are stimulated daily in the best way, especially in the first year, then the foundation is laid for a healthy soul-spiritual self experience with the body and in the body.

Senses oriented to body, soul and spirit

We have twelve senses that can be divided into three main groups. On the one hand, we have the group of body oriented senses – sense of touch, sense of life, sense of movement, sense of balance – and on the other hand the spiritually oriented senses – sense of hearing, sense of speech or word sense, sense of thought, and I-sense (sensing of the other I). Between these we find the soul oriented senses – sense of smell, of taste, of sight and of warmth. All these senses do not work alone but are connected with one another; that is especially the case between the body and the spiritual senses.

– Connection between the sense of hearing and balance

The sense of hearing and the sense of balance are closely connected with each other: If we are not balanced in our soul, we have a hard time listening; for we are completely occupied with our own affairs. We need inner balance which shows itself in form of inner peace and calm, in order to be totally open. The ability to create inner calm and open ourselves to the outside, we owe to the experiences of the sense of balance. That means – and this is decisive – our I, our Self, experiences itself in the sense activity. It is the task, yes, even the meaning of life on earth that the spirit, the I, can experience itself as an individual by bumping into the physical world. This self experience is possible because the mentioned twelve senses are a creation of God, just as we, the whole human being, are wanted by God.

– Connection between sense of word / speech and sense of movement

The sense of movement and the sense of word/speech are connected insofar as every movement that the child learns has a sense-, word-, speech connection: every gesture, every physiognomic expression is speech; every movement is expression of something. The child's future word- and sense experience is decisively promoted through movement development in the first years of life. To the sense of movement we owe our feeling of freedom. If a person feels inwardly free, he can also express himself freely. If not free, he can also not express himself. We can recognize that a person is not free when he always thinks about what he said to whom and when and where. He is unsure and feels many restraints. Persons not free also do not venture into risks, they want to be safe and secure. Freedom of movement changes into freedom of expression. Through freedom of movement, we experience that we, as human beings, are really predisposed for freedom. Only via the sense of movement can freedom become personal experience.

– Connection between sense of life and sense of thought

The same applies to the life processes and thinking. Healthy diet, a good rhythm in life, caring for the life forces are the best ways to further intelligence, the best ways to further the perception of the thoughts and life processes of others. The sense of life brings me into harmony with myself, for it lets me know through hunger, thirst, that something is missing, that I am lacking something. When the need is satisfied, I am content and in harmony with myself. The task of the sense of thought is, to come into harmony with the environment through the effort I make with my thinking. This is encouraged by the sense of life. People who have experienced a certain degree of self-contentment and harmony and this becomes a habit constitutionally, they feel the need to create harmony around them as well. However, anyone who is used to disharmony does not perceive this as a problem. Under certain circumstances such people can really be tactless, like an elephant in a China shop, without noticing that they are destroying the atmosphere and therefore are disrupting connections. The sense of life and the sense of thought are very important social senses. Of course, harmony addiction and over-sensitivity pose another problematic extreme. On the whole, we can say: the ability to experience ourselves as a being of integrity, seeking harmony and capable of it, this we owe to these two senses.

– The Connection between the sense of touch and the sense of I (or sense of the other)

Now the connection between the sense of touch and the I-sense: The most important self experience that the infant has occurs via the surface- and depth sensibility, in that the child feels limits, he experiences, albeit in a dull and unconscious way: I am. We owe the experience that we exist to the sense of touch, it is the basis of a healthy self-awareness, not undermined by doubt in our own existence. If I am convinced of my own existence, I can also develop a sense to perceive other existences. When we cannot perceive ourselves, then we can also not perceive others. Only when the I-sense, which is the sense of perceiving the I of the other, develops undisturbed can social competence develop later on.

Since the child first has to experience himself, the body oriented senses – sense of touch, sense of life, sense of movement and balance – are completely in the foreground during the first year of life. The social senses – The I-sense, sense of thought, of word and of hearing are still closely connected to the body oriented senses in the small child. Rudolf Steiner remarks: What is hidden in the sense of touch reveals itself later in the I-sense, this applies accordingly for the other pairs of senses. When the young child touches the mother or another person, the child touches at the same time their I, their innermost being. He experiences thoughts and words in the harmonious or unharmonious circumstances of life as well as in the gestures and movements of his environment.

The middle senses

Now to the above mentioned middle senses. They let us perceive warmth, light, sound, color, darkness, and various tastes and smells.

- The *sense of sight* makes it possible for us to distinguish light and darkness; we owe to it the optical orientation.
- The *sense of smell* makes it possible that we unite ourselves totally with another being; for whatever we smell, we take it completely into ourselves.
- The *sense of taste* lets us taste not only food but also ourselves or a situation; it is the basis of experience for the later feeling for tact in the soul.
- The *sense of warmth* serves to regulate the body temperature; it is also the basis for our later ability to warm ourselves for something, to become enthusiastic. The development of all these senses moves quickly. If it is disturbed in the first year of life, when all organs but particularly the nervous system, experiences the strongest imprinting, then the child will be predisposed to a more or less severe disability which will hinder a healthy awakening in the body.

In the infant and toddler body, soul and spirit are still intertwined. Spiritual, soul- and physical experiences are still one. The older a human being becomes, the more spirit, soul and body move apart, and each becomes its own area of existence and becomes independent of the others. Then it is possible to endure great soul stress without loss of appetite and insomnia. This must be the case, since in the second half of life the body's resilience decreases, even becomes damaged, and this must not affect the self-esteem. At the beginning of life however, the spirit must awaken in the body and through the body, and the body must facilitate this development by being a support. When the spirit was taken up by thinking and the soul qualities, such as trust in existence, harmony and the experiences of freedom, rest, warmth, light etc., were internalized and are available, then the body can feel badly at times without the affected person falling spiritually out of balance.

Soul-forces and the path of schooling – basis for the development of feeling

The most critical realm of self-experience is the soul life. In thinking I can grasp the ideals of my self wonderfully. But to keep myself upright in my soul between ideal and reality is often extremely difficult. We need to find something that can mediate and do justice to life, so that we do not reject ideals and let ourselves go but that we continue to work on the development of our self-awareness, that we bring with us from our childhood and youth in a more or less stable condition and take with us into life. Especially the soul-life makes it necessary to take a path of development that helps us to trust that out of the environment help will come by affirming, loving and respecting it. The best education is of little use, if it does not turn later into self education. And the consequences of serious deficiencies in education can only be compensated, if a strong personality takes the reins into his/her own hands or if new paths are opened through therapy.

I would like to mention a motive that I think is most important for vocations centering on the young child. Most important is – it was already mentioned above: to practice love. Our feeling life, our soul-life moves in a field of tension between sympathy and antipathy. But there is no place for love in this area; as feeling, as soul reality it does, at first, not exist at all. It is something that every person has to work for. Anyone who confuses sympathy with love, does not know love, and will one day become painfully aware it, when sympathy turns to antipathy. Love can never turn to antipathy. Rather, it mediates between the opposing forces of antipathy and sympathy. The latter belong to the human constitution and are given to us. But love must first be developed, it does not spontaneously appear. Through love antipathy becomes more and more objective and differentiated. To the extend that our ability to love unfolds, antipathy reduces itself more and more to what is actually evil, destructive, and problematic. And the soul sympathies also change themselves, they bring to our consciousness what we perceive as true, beautiful and good.

To develop love means, to work on our sympathies and antipathies so that they become organs of perception that help us to judge objectively and that we can freely make use of. That is the path of schooling of the middle, that above all educators must tread who work with young children. For, when dealing with young children, but also with the parents of young children, there are many natural, instinctual emotions involved: feelings of guilt, envy, anger, suspicion and more. In this muddle we only gain clarity when we work on the cleansing and objectifying of our own soul-life. Only then do we become able, to build up a really healthy and stable self-confidence, and, for instance, can admire someone else without envying him, or condemning something sharply without becoming loveless. For, only when someone feels that he is not hated or rejected, can he accept our judgment. The social competence, and the possibility to really prosper in our work in the social sphere, depends strongly on the education of the feelings through the force love.

The reality of the spiritual-scientific perspective

We can basically assume that when we speak about the body and soul of children and adults there is always something very crucial missing. This brings up images, that hide something because the spiritual point of view does not appear. Most theories are based on the assumption that experiences in early childhood have very definite effects that later determine life; they always only count on *one* earthly life. And even most of the hypnotic techniques that lead back remain in the realm of psychology. If you talk to people who have undergone such retrospectives, or if we read books about rebirthing, we soon realize that certain motives are constantly repeated, especially very specific situations in which the individual was a victim: holocaust, torture, rape, running a spit, being burnt etc., very specific extreme situations of being human. In individual cases this can actually apply.

From Rudolf Steiner's spiritual science, it is known, however, that the human being lays aside his ether body and astral body in life after death. What does that mean? While we take with us thoughts that come from self-awareness and self-experience, from essence and being, we leave behind thoughts of evil, of the perverse, unnatural and abysmal, because they are not part of our being, even if we experienced and endured them. They are not true, beautiful and good. We leave them in the sub-lunar sphere, the sphere between earth and moon. They remain in the etheric aura of the earth and constitute its painful character. In this sphere the demonic, and the evil is at home, the evil thoughts and feelings, the impulses of hate. Now, when human souls approach the earth on their way to rebirth, to incarnation, they perceive many of the fearful cruelties and atrocities in this sphere that happen on the earth. These impressions are included in the forming of the ether body and can emerge in our consciousness as something that we actually experienced. However, it is not our own karma that we are looking at rather, we experience our connection with the karma of humanity, and of humanities guilt, and we want to work in this life on the resolution of it.

The Sistine Madonna as guiding picture of child development

Are there guiding pictures for child development that can help us to find answers to certain questions more easily for the practice?

The Sistine Madonna seems to me to be a basic guiding picture for child development. It is a kind of archetypal Madonna that only Raphael could paint. The German painter Dürer said that with his Madonnas he brought «heaven down to earth».

That she is white-skinned does not mean that she cannot also be archetypal for colored or dark-skinned people. I always recommend that in colored Kindergartens a colored Madonna will be next to this special Raphael Madonna in order not to cause misunderstanding that the white Madonna would be more «normal» than a black one. As color, white expresses in a spiritual sense nearness to God on earth; Black is the esoteric color for death, for spirituality. White speaks of the ideal of purification of the soul on earth, black is the guiding picture of eternity. The human skin-colors can be arranged between these two poles of incarnating and excarnating spirituality.

The Madonna of Raphael is also an archetype in the esoteric sense because her child is neither white nor black but of the color of incarnation, i.e. he mixed into the white some black and red. In black and red the spirituality (the spiritual world) lingers on. Simultaneously, white expresses the will to turn earthwards to show the will to incarnate. This also applies for all the delicate surrounding children's heads. This Madonna picture is esoterically important because seen spiritually, every color and every form is correctly attuned, and the child is placed in such a way on the mother's arm, that the child seems to step forward out of the choir of the unborn, incarnation seeking souls. This is a circumstance that surrounds every young child like an aura: that so many other children, other destinies are in the environment.

A newborn is infinitely rich in lingering experiences from the spiritual world, in etheric ties, hierarchical thoughts but also in karma and destiny connections. This is beautifully expressed by the angel and the male figure who are on the picture besides the Madonna and the child. That is the archetype of esoteric-exoteric composition for the moment of incarnation.

When we have this picture before our eyes and go to work with our infant care in nurseries and crèches, we can gain from this the right attitude and strength, to lead the child in a healthy way on his path to the earth.

From this picture emanates a strong, in the best sense educational, uprightness inspiring, stabilizing force. It is told that people who look at the original of the Sistine Madonna in Dresden, at times stop as if in shock before it and become silent. It is even reported that it took the breath away from a troop of noisy soldiers, who stopped laughing and making jokes.

The gaze of a three-months old child

From developmental psychology but also from personal experience, it is well known, that an infant in the third month begins to fixate people and things with his gaze. Only from this point in time can he really see objects. The complete maturation of the visual faculty to perceive all shades of color, really takes six to eight years. The physiological visual process continues to mature day be day.

At the age of three months, the child also perceives us ever more directly and concretely, and seeks contact with his eyes, with a gaze that seems to penetrate us totally. An infant does not turn his gaze away – with undisturbed calm and steadfastness, we can look into his open, clear eyes. Out of them speaks a spiritual force of love that is objective, full of trust, but also very personal. Only those in love give one another such a comparably long gaze.

Our gazes can touch «etherically»; we notice that in moments when we feel the gaze of another person resting on us – in a good as also in a bad way, for this touching can also come with unclean feelings. A good gaze accompanied by

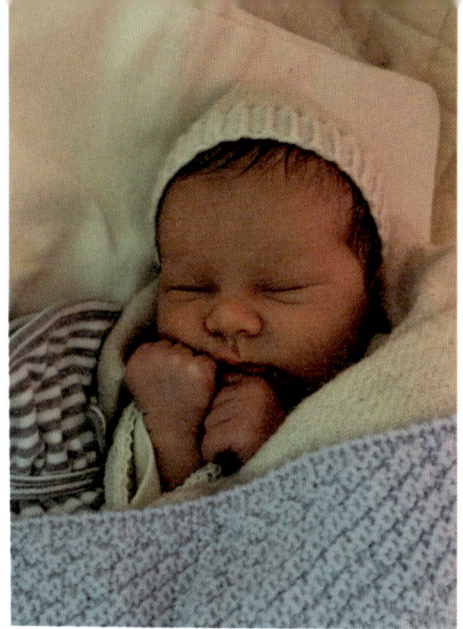
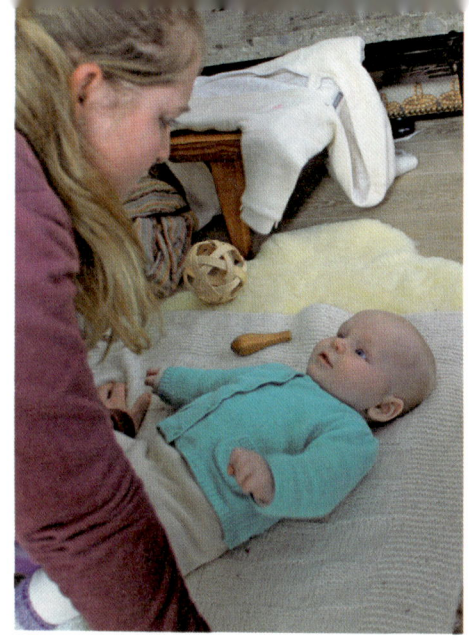

pure feelings can encourage, heal, console and bring light! The ether body – that is, the sum of all the life sustaining lawful processes – can move relatively free from the eye in the intentional direction of the gaze. Seeing is an etheric touching, forming, grasping and molding. The eye muscles help the eye always to move along in the act of seeing. It is actually like an «etheric camera», that we use to touch all sense impressions, and taking them in, imprint them into our thought life. Since we think with the body free etheric life-activity, we can immediately form mental images of all that we see when we close our eyes and remember it.

The gaze of the infant can be a picture for us, how important a pure and honest relationship is. For the child, who looks at us with earnest, trusting gaze studies us and asks:

Are you at my side?
Will you give me what I need?
Can I really trust you? Will you go along with me for some time?

All this lights up before our inner eye, when we meet this earnest, questioning, trusting gaze of the infant. We recognize our task, to become once again so capable of relating to others as we ourselves were as young child – in order not to disappoint this gaze.

Joy and Cheerfulness

Joy and cheerfulness bring about the atmosphere in which the incarnation of a child succeeds best. Rudolf Steiner spoke about that in his lecture, «The Education of the Child, and Early Lectures on Education»:

The joy of children in and with their environment must therefore be counted among the forces that build and shape the physical organs. They need teachers that look and act with happiness and, most of all, with honest unaffected love. Such a love that streams, as it were, with warmth through the physical environment of the children may be said to literally «hatch» the forms of the physical organs. The children who live in such an atmosphere of love and warmth, and who have around them truly good examples to imitate, are living in their proper element. One should not do anything that one would then have to say to a child, you should not do that.[2]

---

[2] Rudolf Steiner, *The Education of the Child and Early Lectures on Education* (A Collection). Anthroposophic Press, 1996.

Christoph Meinecke
The Dignity of Destiny and the Arrival on Earth

«Receiving with reverence, educating with love, releasing in freedom.»
Rudolf Steiner[1]

In the last years and decades, Waldorf pedagogy has dealt increasingly with the first years of life. In many places Waldorf infant care in nurseries and crèches (Waldorfkrippen/Wiegestuben) are beginning. The situation of the families in our society are shaped by the economic life, employment has become a prized asset. We are constantly occupied in Berlin with families who wrestle with the question whether they should put their child into an early day care situation or not.

Higher rates of illness among nursery school children

During a conference of the family network in Germany in 2007 in the city of Mainz with the title «Less State – more parents: What do our youngest children need»? – Professor Hellbrügge from the Children's Center in Munich and Sir Richard Bowlby, one of the leading bonding experts, presented research outcomes concerning infants and young children, who were handed over to child care. Briefly: Children raised early in child care and nurseries show a higher rate of illness. This is not only bad, because as we know, those who have gone through many little infections as child, are developing a strong immune system and later suffer less from e.g. allergies. Unfortunately, far worse illnesses such as meningitis and others appear. The assessment shows in addition, that children in day care show more behavior- and speech-development disturbances than children who were only sent at the age of four into a day care situation.

The researchers found that a feeling of insecurity in relationships and bonding with children in early day care continued often into the third generation. Among day care children there appeared an increase in hearing problems due to the sound volume in that environment. Day care children suffer from elevated stress hormone levels in the blood. We know, that Cortisol and other stress-hormones diminish the plasticity of the brain, and weaken the infection defense and also the frustration tolerance. These children are therefore more disposed to psychic illnesses. It is interesting, that an early day care situation harms boys more than girls.

Waldorf pedagogy in Child Care

In Waldorf circles it was off-limits for decades, to send children into early day care. On the other hand, Steiner already bemoaned that Waldorf education often comes too late because the formative influences happen in the earliest childhood. In his «Study of Man»[2] Steiner expresses his hope that parents may grasp the importance of the first years of life.

As parents, we are faced with the question how we can develop the competence to give the child a healthy and optimal

---

[1] Rudolf Steiner, *Wahrspruchworte. Truth Wrought Words.* GA 40.

[2] Rudolf Steiner, *Study of Man.* GA 293.

space for his/her development. As educators and physicians the question arises of how we can support the parents and family members. Only after that should be considered if additional care persons become necessary to assist the parents or as substitutes.

Both points of view are important when we are dealing with young child pedagogy and the design of nurseries:
- Young children should find there a living space appropriate for them.
- At the same time the family as such should be strengthened.

The path of destiny of the child is respected, if we try to check in each case what is right. Neither the pragmatic decision to give the child away from home early because of parental employment, nor the more dogmatic one, not to give the child away early under any circumstances. In each case, we have to sense what is right for the child. The right decision can only be based on the perception and the feeling what is wanted by the child and his destiny path. Where we experience, after weighing all the details available at the moment, in this case this is the right one.

The fact is that today we are increasingly confronted with the question of early outside assistance. On the one hand, in the above sense, it helps to work together with parents on what they really want. On the other hand, it is very helpful to deepen the understanding of the nature of the child in order to anchor him/her in the hearts of parents, educators and, ultimately, all people. In this sense, I would like to place a few pictures before you.

The path of the human being down to earth

The destiny of a human being unfolds in repeated earth lives. A child that comes to us has already passed through a world of experience before his birth. Rudolf Steiner gives us precise indications: Before the human being comes into this world, he/she experiences a time of retrospect of his previous life:
- In the first third he looks at what he experienced in life, what happened to him and next to him, but also what he could have experienced but did not because he walked past it unconsciously.
- In the second third of the time after death, he looks at all these experiences and «non-experiences» in their significance and consequence for the development of the whole humanity.
- In the last third, the human being experiences the soul-spiritual world that surrounds him, as world of beings. At this point, he has the impulse to come back to earth. He makes the decision to enter into a body again and begin a new life on earth.

Rudolf Steiner tells us how angelic beings, the hierarchies, accompany this path of the human being to the earth and teach him. He now lives deeply immersed in this teaching and forms out of imitation his bodily germ. This experience gives birth to the child's imitative power. Rudolf Steiner tells us succinctly, that we should realize that the children who come to us already have knowledge. They are people, who already have many earth lives behind them. Instead of teaching them, we should try to find out what teachings the children bring with them to Earth.

The task of the educator

In 1921 Steiner addressed the teacher with the following appeal:

> Today we have the task to say to ourselves, the child is educated. It only surrounded the educated soul with a physical body. We have to penetrate this sheath. We must raise up that pre-birth divine instruction ...
>
> ... This is the way we have to think about education today. When we think according to anthroposophic Spiritual Science, it becomes clear, that we cannot do more than remove the hindrances that block what the child brings along from pre-earthly life from revealing itself. That is why in Waldorf pedagogy infinite value is placed on the teacher looking at the child before him as a riddle, that he is asked to solve. Therefore, he should not emphasize instructing the child in something that he has planned, and drum it in. He should never proceed dogmatically but has to see the child himself as his teacher. His task is to observe, how the child tells him through his particular behavior how the sheaths are to be penetrated, so that the divine teaching can emerge from the child. This is the attitude that can move us in the beginning when the children are placed into our arms. The child is an all around complete being.[3]

There is today a large text book with the title: «The Competent Infant.»[4] The little child is a being who already has many talents and a purpose in life. Our task is to create a space where s/he can develop this life purpose.

Universal trust and self-trust

I am fortunate enough to work with newborns. To see with what ease children, who just a few days ago were still hidden from view, now lie in the arms of their parents, fills us with reverence and astonishment. We all have experienced this wonderful time of pregnancy that the children now have directly behind them. Like them, we were warmed in the body of the mother and protected and embraced. We were carried and nourished. From this experience we bring with us the great strength, the strength of universal trust.

We were able to experience that we were cared for, that there was room for us. We had the experience: we were planned. We are wanted.

A motive, in early childhood is gradually to transform these forces of universal trust into forces of self-trust. It helps parents very much to carry this picture in them:

- In universal trust the forces of trust come from the environment. They carry us, are given to us.
- In self trust the forces of trust stream through us into the world. We become active in and for the world according to our life impulse that we brought with us.

---

3   Rudolf Steiner, *Der Mensch in seinem Zusammenhang mit dem Kosmos*. The human being and his connection to the cosmos. GA 203, Vol. 3.

4   Martin Dornes, *Der kompetente Säugling. Die präverbale Entwicklung des Menschen*, Frankfurt/M., 14. ed. 2009. (The Competent Infant)

An important element in preventive parent-work is to awaken the feeling that this developmental process takes time. The child must not be pushed too fast into the rough world, in order not to violate his universal trust. On the other hand, we have to give the space, where s/he can experience himself. This process from universal trust to self-trust, which we call «childhood», takes time.

Places where human beings feel at home on earth

When we come to earth as human beings, we are born into three spheres of life, into three essential destiny worlds that will determine our lives from then on, in which our lives play out and which we must actively cultivate and shape. In these three areas, we must feel at home, to fulfill our life's tasks.

1. Physical home

First and foremost, we must take hold of our own body, our physical home. To arrive well in the body is an essential theme of childhood. When we incarnate well in our body, when we form and build it in a healthy way, it can be a safe instrument for our entire life, and from there our higher spiritual- and soul- forces can develop.

2. Spatial home

The second thing is the spatial home. We look for a certain location: We are perhaps born in Germany or in Switzerland, in Berlin or in Basel. The body, that we select and the location, the spatial environment, belong to our destiny. We need protection in the spatial environment: Clothing, a house, the city, the country, the continent. The development of the human being takes its course in this way, that the living space becomes wider and wider. At first we need a protected home, we need sheaths and the certainty that we have a safe space. From here our horizon widens more and more into the world.

3. Social home

The third destiny connection to which we are bound on earth, we can call «social home». We all need social relationships and connections in life. The child has to arrive on earth in these three places.

(The fourth is the spiritual world. From there the child comes, s/he brings it along. Here in the earthly life, it needs continued care just like the other three.)
To take hold of these three incarnation sites, everyone needs to be involved: The child with his intentions, we the care givers, the parents and educators, all gathered around the child. We prepare the space for him where he can arrive. Rudolf Steiner made wonderful references to these three worlds in the anthroposophic teaching of the senses:

1. Steiner called the objects of perception of the lower senses, connected with the body, the «personal world».
2. The middle senses penetrate the «environment».
3. The upper senses the «social world».

These are the worlds that need to be prepared for the young child.

I: The Lower senses and the personal world

The lower senses help the human being to build up life forces, develop movement etc. We need to ask ourselves:

How can we support the child to take hold of his body?
What hindrances have to be removed?
How can the child remodel the inherited body to create his own?

2: The Middle senses and the environment

How do we prepare the spatial environment for the child? How can s/he learn to perceive the world?
How can s/he develop his senses, experience and understand the world so that later, s/he can work in the world with meaningful actions?

From present day neurobiology we know that a child must learn with all the senses and that this does not succeed via the screen. S/he must be engaged with all senses in learning, must touch, smell, taste. The child wants to become one with the world, would like to sink into the environment with his senses. And therefore, it strongly depends on how we prepare this environment. We have for example, a painting by Raphael on the wall of the room. The eye will execute many more searching movements and this will lead to stronger networking in the brain, than if we have a Donald-Duck figure on the wall, or a light blue elephant. This shows that we affect the learning of the child with the decoration of his environment. In this way we influence enormously how the child takes hold of the world.

3: Upper senses and the social world

The third essential area is the social relationships. Relationships are vital to the human being. Bonding research has produced valuable information about this over the past decades. Already in the first days of life, the child builds up social connections very actively. Only a single caregiver is initially necessary who gives him/her everything needed. Normally that is the birth mother. The interesting thing is that the caregiver could be exchanged in the first few days after birth, but only up to a certain point in time. A later loss leaves a scar in the child's soul, leading to stress and anxiety reactions.

How do we design the bonding structure? What is conducive to building this relationship?

From bonding research we know that the child responds with stress, when we are putting on diapers, clothing or washing him/her, etc., and we are not inwardly present, not in touch, not in relationship with him, but in our thoughts, somewhere else. The heart begins to race, breathing accelerates, the stress hormones in the blood rise.

Relationship needs Communication

Bonding research proves the need to use three main communication tools with the very young child: touch, language, and gaze.

There is e.g. a study that shows that children, who often see positive, radiant faces thrive better. The developmental psychologists call it «Eye greeting» or «Smile-dialogue». We usually do that automatically. We beam at the child when he turns towards us. Rudolf Steiner said that cheerful faces of the educators hatch the child's healthy organs. Today we know that's true. Rudolf Steiner put it this way: «*They need teachers that look and act with happiness and, most of all, with unaffected love … (this) may be said to literally ‹hatch› the forms of the physical organs.*»[5] Today we know this is right.

It is equally important to speak with the child, to tell him what you are doing, and what you will be doing. We should not explain the world to the child, but tell him about it. Children, to whom the world is explained too early, develop fears. I have to mention this to parents, over and over again, during my office hours, especially to fathers. The child cannot yet grasp explanations, that is why they cause fear.

The child wants to learn how the world is. S/he does not want to know at the preschool age, why it is that way. Narratives connect it positively with the world. Rudolf Steiner emphasized numerous times that the child comes into this world with the consciousness: The world is good. He has already experienced in the mother's womb how well everything was prepared. This is the basis for the existential trust. He reads from our gaze, our expression and our speaking that the «world is good».

From linguistic and bonding research we know that factual explanations like «Now we clean the bottom, that it does not get sore», are less fruitful than the speech of «Ammensprache» (speech of a wet-nurse): «Now, I will turn you over on your side, and we will clean your little bottom». We raise the vocal frequency and stretch the syllables a bit. This has nothing to do with baby talk and is exactly what promotes language development and relationship. Equally important is the element of the announcement: The child experiences that it is included and prepared, that mom and dad know what they are doing. This too is a picture that parents can carry in their hearts.

Relationship and Healthy Development

Twenty-year-old students were asked whether as children they felt well cared for by their parents and experienced a warm home atmosphere. The group that affirmed this was found to be 50 percent of the time, less often ill at the age of 50. Relationship, attachment, love are essential preventive elements for a safe and healthy development, not only psychologically but also physically.

To design infant care facilities, nurseries, crèches according to Waldorf pedagogy poses a great challenge, and I myself have the greatest respect for them. In no way should we endanger the attachment to the parents in any way. On the contrary, we should assist the parents in finding ways to optimally form their relationship with the child during the time they have

---

[5] Rudolf Steiner, *The Education of the Child*. GA 34, p. 22.

available. Bonding and relationship arise with time and opportunity.

Developmental steps in the first three years of life

In conclusion, I would like to highlight the three major steps of development of the first years of childhood in two ways:
- learning to walk in the first,
- learning to speak in the second
- and learning to think in the third year of life.

The child acquires these three human abilities completely out of his own volition during the first three years of life. For this development s/he needs a free space. But during this time he is also still guided, he is drawing from forces that he brings along from the prenatal world. Rudolf Steiner describes that the child has the strength for uprightness, for placing himself between cosmos and earth, from the pre-earthly contact with the Archai, the spirits of personality, the time-spirits. The ability to walk, we human beings owe to the teaching of the Archai. In a similar way, we owe the ability to learn to speak to the teachings of the Archangels, the Archangeloi, and the ability to learn to think to the teaching of the Angeloi, the Angels.

But the child also seeks the role model of the adult human being on earth. Rudolf Steiner emphasizes, how important it is that a corresponding moral attitude can be experienced in the child's environment. That fits in with our approach:

Movement development must not happen under duress but should happen out of the joy of movement in full freedom. The child must not be pushed. He does not need development programs, but free areas to develop. According to Steiner, in order to be healthy, the child needs
- to learn to walk, an atmosphere of love and freedom,
- to learn to speak, truthfulness in the language of the teacher,
- to learn to think, clarity in the thinking of the educators.

Christ in the Human Being

In learning to walk, learning to speak and learning to think, according to Steiner, the higher I of the human being, and the power of Christ are at work as forces from which the child draws in the beginning of his life. «To recognize the forces that are effective in a person during childhood is to recognize Christ in man.»[6]

In the first three years of childhood, these forces work without any effort on the part of the human being. The child does not need a plan, in order to accomplish his developmental task. He just does it.

It is comforting: Also in later years these forces can still work in us, when the human being seeks the Christ within himself. Even if not everything went optimally in the first years, not all is lost. Adults and educators who care for the forces of thinking, of speech and of action during the day appropriately can connect during the night with the spheres of the hierarchies:

---

[6] Rudolf Steiner, *The Spiritual Guidance of the Individual and Humanity.* GA 15.

- Regarding thinking, Steiner says: If our thinking was penetrated during the day with idealism and spirituality then in sleep we can link up with the Christ forces working in the Angeloi, and in this way receive forces of healing.
- Concerning the speaking with one another during the day, he says: «*An idealistic, positive attitude towards the other human being concerning speech*» will give speech the richness that would help us during the night to connect with the sphere of the Archangeloi.
- For our deeds and actions the following applies: «*Warm, considerate acts out of respect for others as spirit-beings*» during the day will make it possible to connect during the night with the sphere of the Archai.

These are the three main healing sources of the etheric working of Christ. By practicing these above mentioned abilities, we will acquire the power of love, of respect, of recognition and appreciation for the other person.

Examples of Personal Experiences

In conclusion, I would like to describe two short experiences with children from the recent past, when their wisdom became clear:

A four-year old child, who had never seen me before, hopped joyfully into my office, straight towards me, shook my hand, jumped on the examination bench and said: «I know you, you were also one». Then I could sense, that the search for social destiny connections is universal and always goes beyond one's one family. A more beautiful proof for the existence of the spiritual world and of our pre-earthly being, is hard to imagine.

Another boy, two years of age, had taken a truck during the pre-examination and wanted to leave the room with it. The parents warned me, «He will not give it back». I quickly noticed that the boy really had decided to hold on to the truck. The parents wanted to distract him and gave him a fire truck – without success. Suddenly, a sense of evidence flashed up in me, that the boy wanted to reestablish order. Because the truck belonged in the next room. So, I opened the door and went with him into the next room. Without hesitation he put the truck down and came back upright and satisfied to his parents, who had watched the scene speechlessly.

We can always observe that children have a sense for order and rightness but we often do not give them enough time, to rectify something.

Michaela Glöckler
Autonomy of the young child

Young children are pretty much «autonomy-miracles». If we do not disturb them, they act completely out of themselves, perceive intensively – are totally who they are – only, they do not know it. The reflective self-consciousness that would guide their behavior consciously, has not yet awakened. When we watch an artist at work, we experience a conscious and unconscious autonomously active person. That is the reason, why we bring the art into movement, into speech, into music, but also into the handling of form and color. In the forms, colors, sounds, words and movements certain laws come to expression. Art follows its own laws, as also the sense-perceptible world has its laws. Autonomy does not mean lawlessness. Rather it signifies a sovereign, self-active, creative working with conditions and laws (Greek: «To give laws oneself»). Autonomy is the ability to work in a self-directed way with objects and transform them. To give an example: The letters in the alphabet are very limited. There are languages that have more consonants, others are more reduced in their alphabet – but the amount of letters is always manageable. With these few letters, however, world literature is written and formed, billions of documents! Goethe formulated it this way, that only the law, the condition can give the human being the consciousness of freedom.

Autonomy of the Adult
I had a personal autonomy-shock at age 18, when I was allowed to get my driver's license. The driving instructor was of the opinion that women do not belong behind the wheel, and tried to spoil my attempt at learning to drive with his unpleasant behavior. Today we would call his conduct «mobbing». When I experienced such treatment, seemingly did everything wrong all the time and was laughed at with quite some cynicism, it suddenly became clear to me that as soon as I had the driver's license I could drive wherever I wanted – the circumstances of getting the driver's license did not matter.

Infants cannot talk to themselves like that. Infants and young children cannot distance themselves inwardly from a negative look or a hate-filled gesture. Young children are victims of learning conditions that limit their autonomy. Therefore, the interaction with artistic-means is a decisive schooling for everyone who wants to acquire the competence, to create suitable developmental conditions for another human being.

That means, to bring general laws to effectiveness in such an individual way that the other person can experience himself as autonomous in his activity.

Loss of Autonomy
During our plenum activity, we ask kindly not to take photos in the hall. This has two reasons: Flashlights disturb just like the ringing of cell phones. Even though flashlights are more harmless than the electro-smog of the cell phones, they nevertheless interrupt the quiet, the attention and concentration. If we leave out the moral aspect of lack of respect, a damage of the will occurs that the adult can, how-

ever, compensate. We can clearly observe what happens inwardly, when such an interruption occurs. There are always three stages:
1. We are startled and interrupted.
2. We experience a brief annoyance, and thinks a few dumb things that perhaps we even say.
3. We calm down again and enter anew into the on-going presentation.

We should diagnose such behavior as an expression of loss of autonomy of the modern person. Someone who disturbs is not autonomous but suffers from a strong self-focus. Self-focus is not equal to autonomy. The human self is not an egoist but is the center for our personal development. Personal-development means, in addition to the acquisition self awareness and of social competence, gaining the ability to accomplish deeds within a greater context. For this, an individual development component is necessary: personal commitment, which means to be able to be alone as well as being able to get together with many.

About the Autonomy of the young Child

During the years of my pediatric activity, I met the autonomy of the young child in three different variations. This touched me deeply every time.

1. Penetrating to the Essence

I had the first decisive experience during routine check-ups for infants. I experienced that newborns or those of a few weeks or of two or three months, can gaze with their eyes infinitely deep. When we return that gaze, we experience penetrating to the essence of a being. We experience, how a strong personality wrestles to bring himself to expression in this little body, step by step, and year by year, always a bit better. This personality radiates through the gaze infinitely trusting, and seeks the gaze of the other. When this gaze, this intention is not returned, it retreats again. It is a force breaking through from inside, a pure etheric touching. When looking, the ether-body, our forming force organization, passes through the physical eye to the object of observation. Seeing is an etheric touching, etheric taking hold of. That is why we have this magical experience of being-looked at – an experience that is familiar to all of us, even when we are looked at intensively by a person from the side or the back: we feel it, even though we do not see the other person. Gazes are realities, etheric touch realities. When I look at someone, then my own I moves with intention and with feelings (cold or warm gaze) on the waves of the etheric to the other person. The child immerses himself with his gaze there, and both are weaving in this beholding of each other, in the penetration of each other's being. Adults can only endure that when they are in love. Most of the time, you only look briefly, and then you lowers the gaze again. We cannot endure this strong force, this closeness. We end the process. Children do not end it because they have love and trust. We adults need and must learn, to look at children with objective love, so that the words by

Goethe become true that he wrote to Charlotte von Stein during his love relationship: *I felt good in your eyes.*[1]

The space into which we welcome young children especially in the first and second year of life, has to be designed in such a way that the children feel well on all levels:

1. physical level: via the senses,
2. etheric level: via the gaze, the relationships, the connections,
3. astral level: via the feeling, how we are in tune emotionally.

This place is like an eye that looks at the child. Not only our eyes, everything out in the environment looks at the child. The more conscious and loving it is designed, the better the child feels, the more welcomed he can experience himself.

2. Doing it oneself

The second experience, that revealed to me something fundamental concerning the autonomy of the young child occurred in the rush of the office hours: a mother wanted remove her child quickly from the consulting room and began to put on his jacket and button it. The child was about two years old. I still see his face today – it was like an initiation, a real wake-up-experience. The child said with a pained face and yet full of good will: «do it myself». While the mother buttoned, he whaled impatiently again and again: «Do it myself».

It became clear to me, how many things in daily life we do for each other, that perhaps the other person would have preferred to do himself. This does not just apply to children. We can also annoy an adult, by mothering him too much and thinking that you constantly have to do something for him, constantly have to perform. It is about giving the other some space and only intervening when it is necessary. When we ask, the autonomy is maintained. However, the autonomy of the other is also preserved, when the other person for whatever reason, needs help or – as in the case of the child – the time is pressing, and we are conscious of our infringement when acting. Then our action will be experienced differently than if the awareness was not there. When the child experiences the possibilities to act himself as something arbitrary – at times I may at other times not –, he does not experience in our actions any logic. But when we excuse ourselves and say – «Mama will quickly button the jacket now so we can leave, but at home you may do it again» – then the child feels respected in his autonomy.

3. Assisting self-help

The third experience was the observation, how very young children are dependent on the inner attitude of adults concerning their autonomous will to learn and create. This immense dependence is obvious already when cutting the cord after birth. The child is cut off from the mother. S/he is detached from her but in dire need of help. Maximum help is necessary for self-

---

[1] Johann Wolfgang von Goethe, *Warum gabst du uns die tiefen Blicke*. In: Sämtliche Gedichte. Berlin 2007. (Why did you cast such deep gaze on us)

help to develop, maximum support to develop autonomy. That is the greatest contradiction: In the first year of life, the human being is least accessible to indoctrination and learning programs of any kind. He is totally autonomous – and yet s/he is in most need of help. In face of this need for help, we can learn best, how to help children become autonomous at the beginning of their lives.

I would like to point out in the form of a five-star, which basic attitudes and qualities we need as adults, in order to help the child to develop his autonomy – and thereby also develop our own further. But before that, a comment on what happens when autonomy can not develop well.

We observe e.g. in case of severe personality disorders and in case of illness autonomy deficits. For example, the so-called borderline disorder is a widespread psychiatric disease. It has been found that a person with a borderline personality behaves very differently in different situations, depending on which person he is with. Of course, this applies a little bit to each of us, but especially for a borderline – personality. He *is* then really different when he is together with someone else. His counterpart feels well understood and thinks, that they spoke together wonderfully, but afterwards, one cannot rely on anything that was said. It has been found that the causes for the borderline-disorder go back to the first three years of life, especially to the first and second years of life.

The Human Being as a Pentagram, with his five essential qualities

- The «left foot», the «Standbein», represents the physical body.
- The «right foot», the «Spielbein», represents the etheric body.
- The «left arm» represents the astral body, and our capacity for empathy.
- Our ego-organization is represented through the «right arm».
- The « head» holds the place for our spiritual orientation, that part of us that is spiritually active beyond the confines of the body.

Note: In sculpting human forms, the terms Standbein and Spielbein refer to the technique of showing a person standing firmly on one leg (the Standbein), with the other leg (the Spielbein) lightly bent, ready to move in any direction.
The star-form of the human being is constructed in such a way that the different «bodies» (Wesensglieder) come to expression in the various regions of the body with different strengths.

1. Physical Aspect – the Spatial body: Playing field for building and designing

When we ask, what we can do from the physical side to protect autonomy, it will be about the wonderful, often very concrete «giving – space». For, the physical body is a spatial body.

2. Etheric Aspect – the time-body: Patience and Mindfulness

With the etheric, we can form processes in time consciously. We should not end them abruptly and in this way, trigger a lesser or stronger shock. It is about consciously handling processes, rhythms, and other time sequences so that transitions, that is, beginnings and endings of actions become possible. Then the child can finish one thing in peace, before another begins and in this way experience himself as master over these processes.

3. Astral Aspect – giving space in the Soul-realm: Joy in the other

It is especially important to accompany the child in a warm, loving way, to open one's soul, to let him/her come, to expect them. Here it is about the giving of soul-space and enveloping. This shows as joyful interest in the child, I communicate: «I am looking forward to you, how are you today»? Intentional joy is another word for interest.

4. I/Ego aspect – building identity: Self-awareness

When children are able to do much by themselves, they will first learn through imitation and later from their «mistakes». In this way the I can experience itself and also feel free. A good educational method creates a path for later self-education.

5. Aspect of spiritual Orientation: Concern for the World, Trust

The best furthering of the autonomy of the child by a spiritually designed environment, is the deep trust of the educators in the guidance of their own destiny and their own path. Without trust, spiritual life is sterile and cannot blossom. Rudolf Steiner wrote a meditation concerning trust in thinking.

In his book «The Threshold of the Spiritual World»[2], he answered an objection that he himself posed, that particularly as far as thinking is concerned, there is a strong distrust: if we did not trust in our thinking as our spiritual competence so completely, we would not pay so much attention to our doubts.

For why do our doubts bother us so much? Because we trust that they could be true, because we do trust our thinking in every situation in life.

Wholeness and Autonomy

Movement is always self-movement and represents wholeness. We saw that in the example of Christoph Meinecke. Movement processes occur always in a certain context. The autonomous self, is a wholeness. This comes best to expression in the wholeness of the movement process: During all of the early childhood development, certain movement patterns are produced by the whole body. The more holistic they can develop, the less interference happens, the more autonomous they become.

Thomas Fuchs, a very well-known neurophysiologist and family therapist in the city of Heidelberg, wrote a great book with the title: «The brain, an organ of relationships»[3]. He summarizes the modern neu-

---

[2] Rudolf Steiner, *Die Schwelle der geistigen Welt*. 1. Kapitel, Aphoristische Ausführungen. GA 17. Berlin 1913. (Road to Self-knowledge)

[3] Thomas Fuchs, *Das Gehirn – ein Beziehungsorgan. Eine phänomenologisch-ökologische Konzeption*. Stuttgart 2010. (The brain, a relationships organ – a phenomenological-ecological concept)

rological research in this way: A person has a brain, but s/he is not that brain.

The brain as organ of relationships, as an instrument, is formed and designed through the way in which the person makes contact with space, process, objects, and beings.

The following questions may accompany today's work:

What is the human I?
What is the principle of autonomy?

Master Ekkehard formulated the beautiful verse: «*If I were a king and did not know it, I would not be a king.*»

We are all meant to be autonomous beings but because we know so little about what autonomy signifies, we are not really autonomous. We can become autonomous to the extend that we bring the principle of autonomy to our consciousness.

Aiming to go one's own path

In conclusion, I would like to demonstrate something. When we look around us today, we see dependency on drugs, on persons, on science, on sexuality, on nutrition. The dependency potential is growing exponentially and is accompanied by a correspondingly low level of autonomy. The Deficit in autonomy and the dependency potential are congruent.

Interesting is, that the foundation for independence is dependent on how children learn to walk. The first year of life is the time where we place ourselves on our own feet. This process is the archetypal picture of becoming independent. When children gladly stand on their own feet and can attain unimpeded freedom of movement we lay the ground for sovereignty and independence for later life.

Once, when I accompanied a drug-dependent person, I learned that a dealer recognizes his clients by their walk. I had asked her why she was approached and offered drugs again and again, yet it never happened to me. She could only laugh: «You know, we recognize each other by our walk».

After that I began to observe walking habits.

What does a gait look like when a dealer recognizes that it is worth addressing the one or the other?

- One way would be that the various members of the human being are too deeply incarnated and the person looks like s/he could start kicking and fighting any moment.
- Another way would be that the members of the human being incarnate too loosely caused by shock, by trauma, or assaults – which causes a slightly flitting, or tripping gait.

Those who walk in a centered, goal oriented way are not approached by dealers.

Last night, the disunity and turmoil of people in our present time was shown by a modern piece of music by Noèmi Böken. The separate parts are held together by experiencing them through Eurythmy and in this way releasing them from their one-sidedness. Interestingly, immunological research has found that intentional, goal-oriented walking stimulates the immune system. Walking in a goal-oriented way for 20 minutes every day is the best immune stimulant. That's why the way we learn to walk can be the most important health care: We should not disturb children's purposefulness and their urge and curiosity to move without any urgent need, in order not to weaken their immunity.

Claudia Grah-Wittich
The Autonomy of the young Child
Examples from the practice

A mother comes with her child for a consultation and is desperate because the boy is not at all stimulated to do anything by himself, although he is four years of age. When she comes home with him, she says: «Take off your shoes, take off your jacket, go wash your hands», he sits and looks at her with big eyes. At first, I had no idea where I could begin. It was intuitive that I asked: «How did your child learn to walk?» Not knowing what I caused, she answered: «That was the best time. He always stretched out his hands to me. I took them and then we practiced walking».

The cause for the behavior of the child now became clear and I could say: «This is what your boy still wishes! He experienced so much joy in you when you took his hand, why should he now walk alone?»

This example shows us, when it is decided whether a child enjoys being by himself and conquering the world in an experimental and autonomous way – or not.

Create opportunities for autonomous development

In this contribution I would like to show, how we can create opportunities in facilities when dealing with the child under the age of three that their autonomy can develop optimally. I will show some pictures, and I would like that we really enter into them so that they may begin to speak to us in the sense of Goethe.

In order to create good opportunities in a facility that children can move autonomously we need to ask:

What does the child want to learn? What is the child already able to do? What kind of opportunities does he need to continue to practice intensively?

I focus on what the child would like to practice and what it already can do. The greatest hindrance to perceive a child, is our own fear. I have been able to observe the daily activities in many facilities. When I asked: «Why do you not let the child do this himself?», the answer is: «For fear that something might happen.»

I must look at two things: To the child and his needs and to myself. I must reflect and find where my fear is located. When I recognize my fear, I already have got hold of the little devils in me, and it will become easier for me to turn to the child and permit development. I am building in this way a kind of sheath around the child in which he can learn by himself.

The knowledge of the body

In the first picture we see Mathilda. She is one and a half years old. She can walk and go down the stairs by herself. The stairs are safe and the environment is prepared. She adjusts well. What can we see?

One foot is firmly placed on the step of the stairs. The other foot, comparable to the «Spielbein» (right leg) of a sculpture, seeks and feels the depth.

How much does she have to adjust the body to the gravity, in order to find the next step well and safely? How deep does the distance feel that she sees?

Look to her hands. The one hand is a little further up on the rope than her head. The other hand is about where the other leg is.

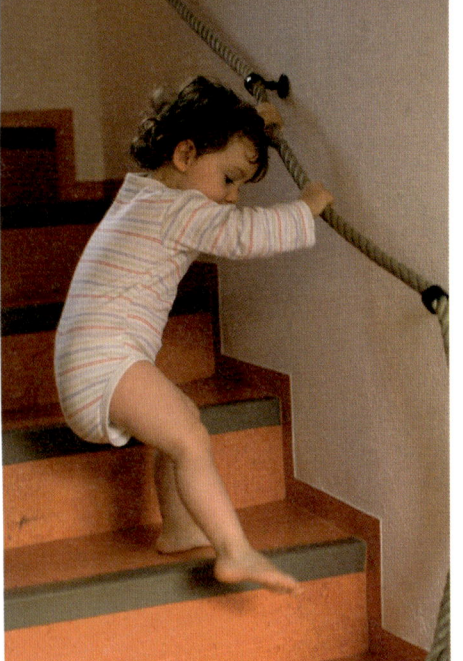

Fig. 1

She secures herself with both hands on the rope. The weight placed upwards on the steps. All skiers and hikers know that it is safer on the slope, when we lean towards the slope and not towards the valley. Mathilda does not need ski instruction, also not stair climbing instruction. Her body already had that knowledge. It is a small miracle. I feel right away, how warmth and joy appear, and they of course, form a sheath for the child. A child that is not disturbed knows how much time she needs for such a learning sequence, and also how often she must try and feel her way. Naturally, this knowledge is not in the head but in the limbs. Mathilda knows in her legs and hands, in her total physiological constitution how she needs to hold on, in order not to lose her balance. Holding the balance is one of the most instable moments for us human beings. Safety for the child, but also for us as parents or educators only arises when we can create it inside independently.

Observation provides trust

Mathilda stands firmly on her left leg, secures herself and feels with her right leg carefully the next step. She is looking with utmost concentration. She is completely in herself. She is at one with herself, the stairs and the process. She directs her gaze to the steps of the stairs and she will slowly place her foot on the next step. A child can give such total attention to this moment only because an adult is close by and accompanies her venture. The attention and concentration of us adults, our backing is like slipping into those feet and hands – and in this way gives us trust also. It is clearly countering the anxious questions whether the child can really make it, whether something might happen. With careful observation you can see by Mathilda's feet and hands whether they are secure. Our attending perception and alertness is an appropriate sheath for Mathilda's efforts.

An important consequence of such a staircase sequence is that Mathilda had the experience of taking on responsibility herself. She does not look for help in her environment but she secures herself.

What does it mean for the rest of a person's life when we have learned such a lesson so early?

The parents' fear is a hindrance

The preliminary stage for such a safe up and down the stairs in a facility or a parent home occurs already much earlier. The following picture comes from a parent-child-group. These groups exist to clear away hindrances between parents and their children, especially also the hindrance of the fear of the parents. When a child crawls down from such a platform as in the picture, head first, supported by the hands, it can happen that the arm cave in because of the weight of the head. Parents think they must quickly jump to help, so that the head does not hit the floor. This overhasty intervention precludes that the child can get a feeling for the depth and his weight. In order to develop the body consciousness, a muscle build-up must take place in the upper arms and in the neck area. Since the development proceeds form the head to the feet, we find the muscle build-up first in the arms and then in the legs. Later the children will turn around all by themselves. The platform is a great support and an ingenious help to give children the chance to become self-sufficient when dealing with heights and depths.

A connection to the environment

Ole has play stairs in a parent-child-group. He can raise himself up at the edge of these play stairs. He stands with his left leg and lifts his right leg slightly to take the next step and climb the first step of the play-stairs (see Fig. 3 on p. 58). In the next picture, he is up on the second step. Now something decisive happens: Ole seeks the gaze of his mother.

The gaze is an invisible touch-reality. We recognize that the ether body of the child has not yet cut the cord. Ole seeks the gaze of his mother who nods to him and affirms with this nod the connection. The invisible «umbilical cord» can be experienced. We meet here a mother who

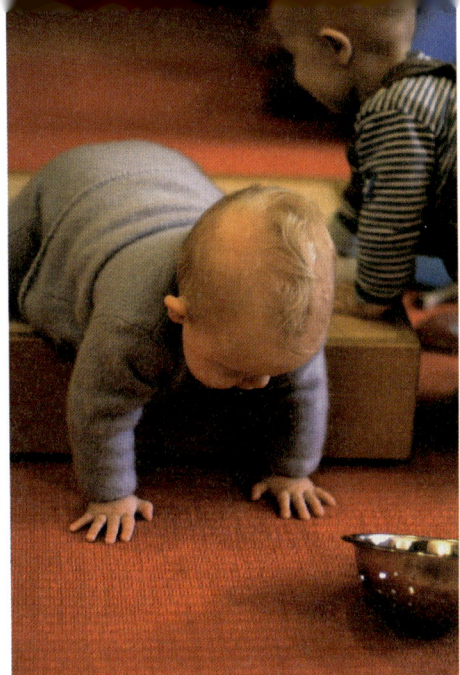

Fig. 2

has practiced. She probably says, «Ole, you are on the second step, if you want, you can come down again. Or you can go further up». This mood is expressed in such communing. It gives the child a feeling of security: «You are right, you practiced. You can continue.» This agreement creates a sheath around the child and the adult. On the next picture: Ole can find the way down by himself. In these examples you see very clearly, how we can study the human being. The children show us: «Yes, this is how it is. We are autonomous beings, but we need the umbilical cord. We need the etheric touch-reality in the gaze as security.» This is shown by this important sequence.

I am skeptical, when there is much crocheting, knitting, cooking and baking, because our attention is distracted, when it is continuously needed by the children. We need to accompany the children in their movement, and therefore play a big part in whether they feel secure or not. There are

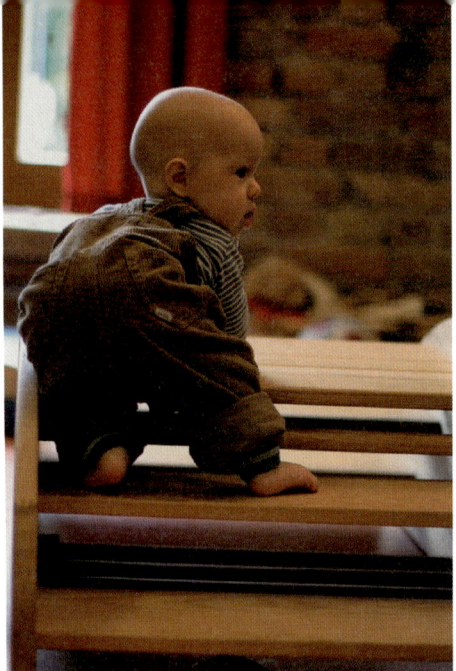 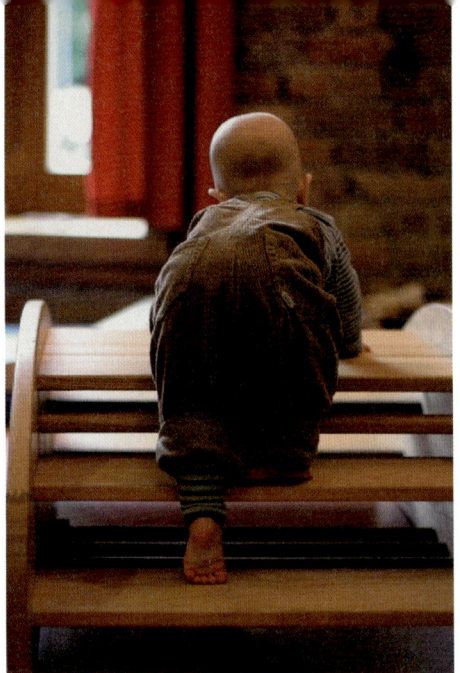

Fig. 3   Fig. 4

many activities in house and garden that we can engage in and at the same time observe them and be there for them, when they need us. We should examine ourselves:

Am I awake in perceiving the children, even when I am active?

That is important, especially when they should develop in a self-sufficient way.

Holistic process

We come to a small series of pictures of Anna. Anna can cope with some stairs in the outdoor area. The stone steps are hard and pointed. For a moment we ourselves, doubted whether we built them properly. Anna makes the doubt disappear quickly. She will now take the first step of the stairs. She stretched on the steps of the stairs, now she is drawing herself together again.

I would like to connect here with Michaela Glöckler's contribution. It is clear that every process is something of a totality, because all etheric – and these are etheric movements – strives for harmony. This striving for harmony becomes visible, when a child executes a contraction after an expansion, as was visible in the stretching of herself and then the drawing together again on the steps of the stairs. In this rhythmic process not only the physical body forms itself but connected to it, also the etheric constitution. In the one picture, Anna's body is pulled together. She looks up, eyes her goal. Now she stretches herself again. She wants to go further up. On the next picture, she pulls together again, prepares for the next expansion. On the following picture she has successfully reached the top.

Pauses are part of it

Do we actually know how it is when we have arrived at the top and it does not go further?

Again, a new situation. What does Anna do in this situation, infinitely knowledgeable in her childhood? Rest! Pause!

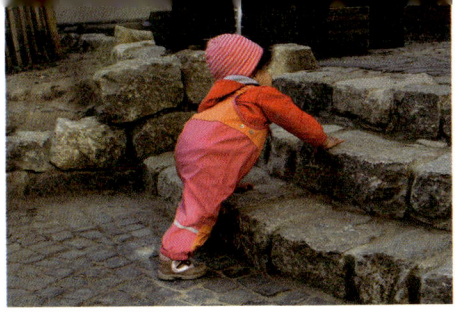
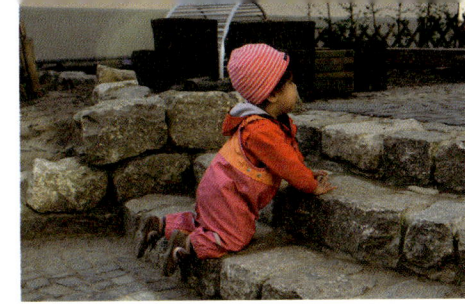
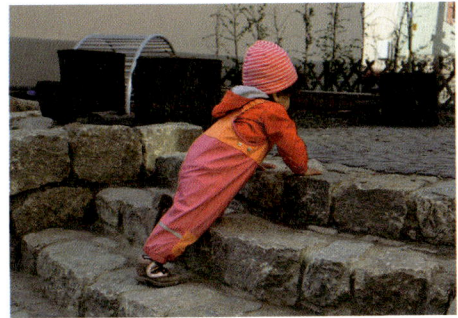
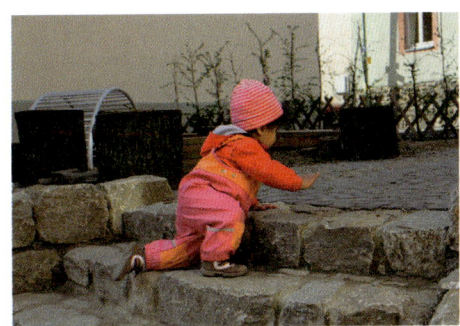
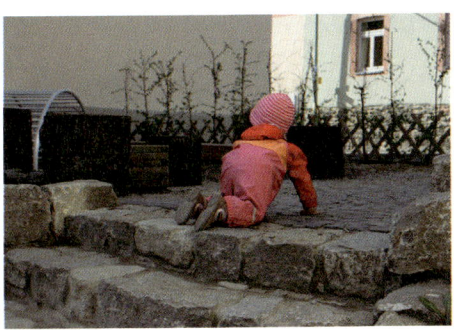
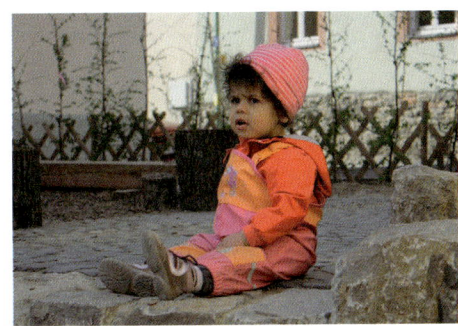

Again a law of the living, of development: there must be a pause. Children know this. They make a pause again and again before they go into a new expansion process.

After the break, Anna moves down the steps again – head first (see picture on p. 60). I do not ask now if or who worries because of this. Look how Anna solves going downwards on the stone steps: She arrives on the top step and notices that it does not go on. She begins to turn herself on the step into a side position and completes this work of art turning herself and pausing again. This resembles an artistic formation, a choreography following wise laws. After a break she continues on, till she reaches the bottom.

Anna shows out of her body-knowledge, the innate knowledge, an artistic, etheric-physical visible formation. She forms herself in this stair-climbing, and achieves in the process a very fine security.

Observing such processes is important for us. If we succeed in this, a deep reverence awakens for these kinds of sequences in child development. Then we can let the children do, and need not constantly interfere. Our fear disappears.

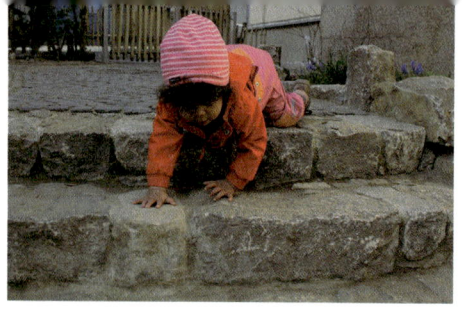
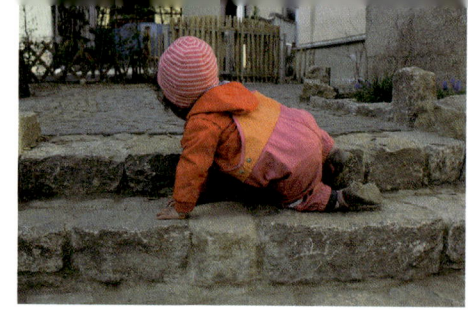
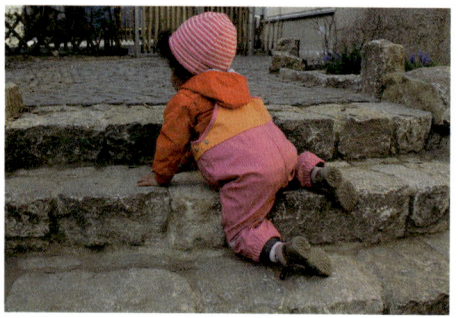

A time for experiments

In other pictures children of different ages present us with varying solutions when mastering stairs. They are artist and manage in a very individual way. Malik, Johanna and Luca normally go backwards down the stairs, crawling on all four. These are very steep stairs in our old farm-house. The teacher went ahead of them. She is now at the bottom, watching and accompanying the children.

- Johanna made an autonomous decision today. She wants to try it differently. She sends the little ones ahead. The teacher says: «Johanna, I guess you want to try to walk today»? Johanna gets all the time she needs to complete this experiment.
- Malik, two-and-a-half years old choses another solution to go downstairs – he slides on his behind.
- Emilio, just two years old, shows how you can slide down the stairs on the knees. When you have children of different ages, then you will most likely have many ways how to accompany children to go down the stairs. Emilio takes much time. He is thorough.
- Then we see a playful variant. When children feel self assured, they can address situations in a playful way.

These were children almost three years of age that will enter Kindergarten soon. They begin to free-style the event out of an inner feeling of self-assurance. They play, they can become creative on the basis of

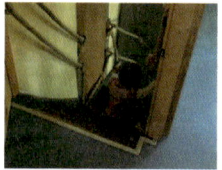
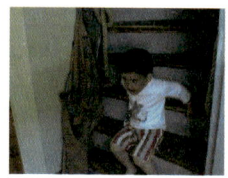
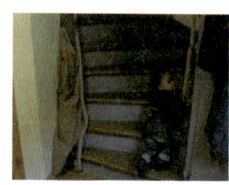
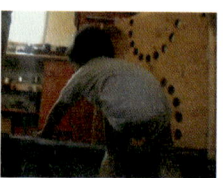

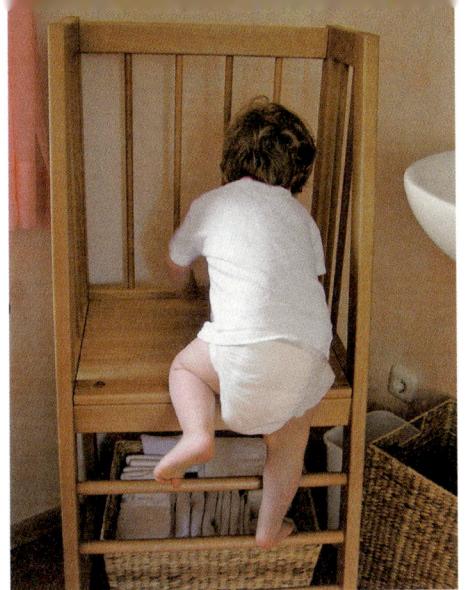 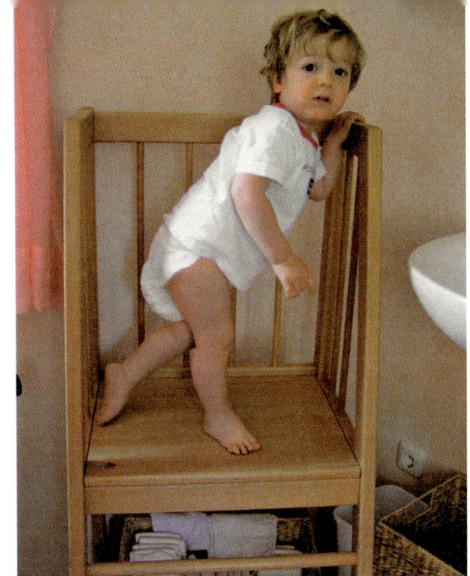

feeling secure. They say: «Today we will go up the stairs like little bugs». Working in early education with children who need support for their development, we are well aware how important it is for these children to come up with such a variety of movements themselves.

Possibilities of educating for autonomy

I would like to show a few pictures of another opportunity to get moving in every day life. In our facility there is a diaper changing table, the somewhat older children may climb up that structure, if they are able. You see how Stefano is climbing up this diaper changing table by himself. You can see him hooking his feet on the steps and holding on in the back. Now he pulls up his knee slowly onto the surface. That is really hard work. Do you think you need to assist? Can he make it? Now he is on top and you still see the effect of gravity: Everything goes downwards but the head is slowly rising. The last picture shows a dancer. He stands up there with great elegance! He made it all by himself. On this changing table he can stand and

have his diapers changed, and can meet the person on eye level that cares for the area where he is not yet self sufficient.

In conclusion, let us treat ourselves to a situation with children who already were in our facility for longer time («Wiegestube»). These children were very autonomous in their movement development but were accompanied there professionally and with much awareness. They are in our garden at a play structure. A play structure is an environment that we offer to the children in order to develop themselves on their own. There is also a swing where the feet touch the ground. The girl has already learnt to swing by herself. It is amazing to see what children can do who earlier had the opportunity to be accompanied in a protected space (see pictures on p. 62).

I would like to encourage you to go back into the every-day life of your facilities with these pictures before your eyes, to see how you can create opportunities for the children, but also for the co-workers to gain more autonomy. For, this topic does not only concern children but all of us.

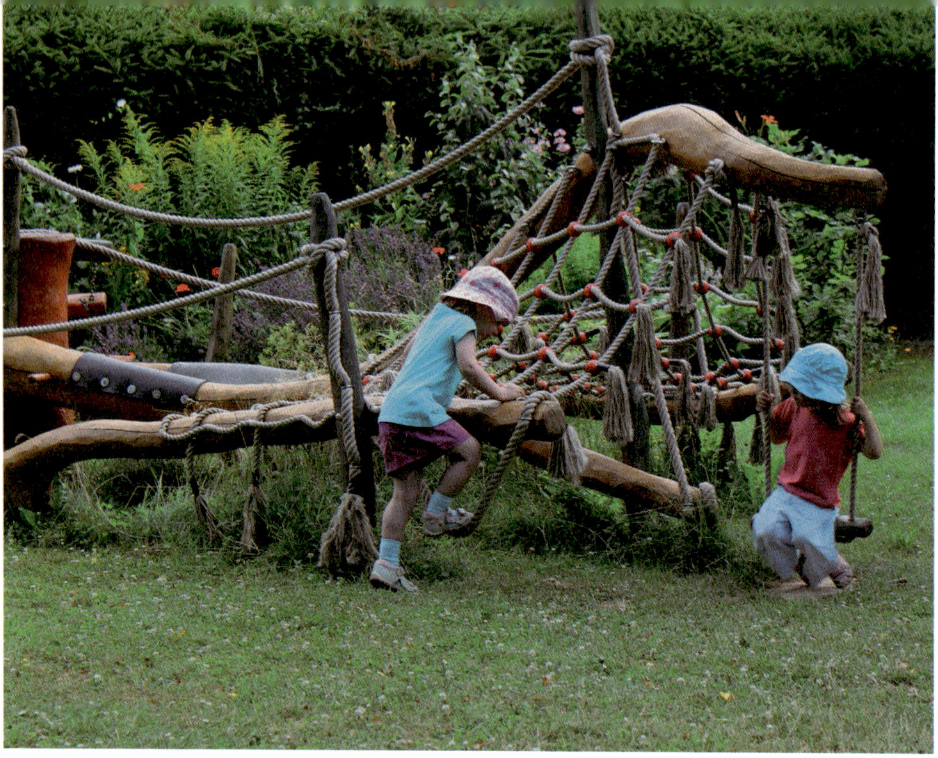

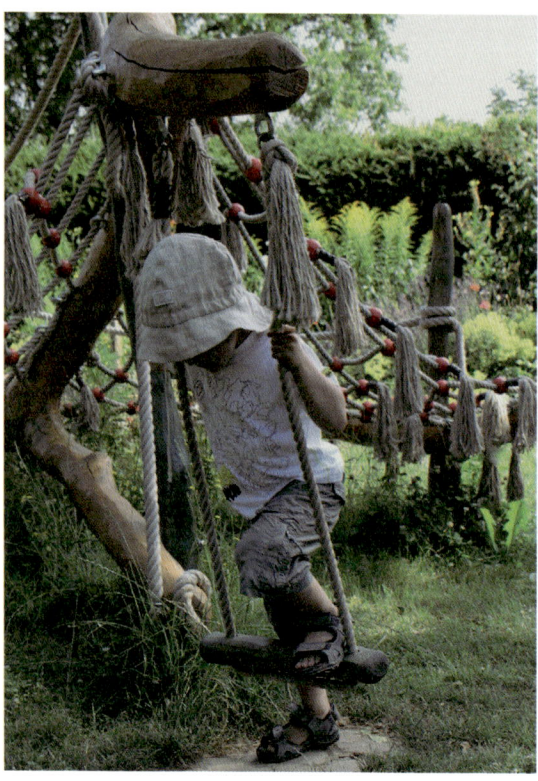

Michaela Glöckler
Concerning the culture of relationships

Our topic this morning concerns the culture of relationships.
When and how does the forming of relationships become a culture?
In cultural history, it was a special moment when in 2008 the «UNO-Convention on the Rights of Persons with Disabilities» came into force, which has since been ratified by 100 states. People with disabilities should be awarded the same basic- and human rights as the so-called non-disabled. The main consideration was, that people with disabilities make a significantly bigger contribution – and now you will be amazed! – to the humanization of humanity. It was not Anthroposophists who said that, they do like to use the term «humanization», but UNO representatives, the designers of the «Convention on the Rights of Persons with Disabilities», they were the ones who said that. This opened a new chapter in empathy and communication. But one might also ask why this was only possible now.

How does empathy, gratitude, a sense of compassion develop?
The speaking and communicative level is close to our feelings and all that is connected with the feelings. We quickly get angry, for instance, we go out of ourselves a bit, when the words are not chosen in such a way that we feel ourselves understood. To take into consciousness this whole soul landscape of speech and communication and use it pedagogically in early childhood education, poses an especially great challenge.

Speech acquisition and Behavior
Why is that so important? In his opening speech, Christoph Meinecke made it clear that speech can have an hurtful effect if it is not benevolent and of goodwill, with a respectful attitude towards the other.

In today's research, which deals with the analysis of rampages, violent crimes and, in general, with the increasing global violence of our society, we are increasingly coming to the conclusion that violence and speech development are closely linked. We speak of «Nonviolent Communication»[1] as well as of a communication that promotes violence. This is pictorially differentiated in the terms «giraffe communication» and «wolf communication». Researchers have found that juvenile criminals, in particular, often have only the level of fourth-grade students, which means, a much smaller, less differentiated ability to express themselves or less vocabulary than other youth. When adults communicate with young children during the time they learn a language, that is, in their vulnerable pre-I-conscious phase, with a negative, punitive, repellent, rejecting attitude, then the children take deeply into themselves that the way of communication is aggressive. The child learns figuratively: If you want to tell another person

---
[1] Non-violent Communication is a concept developed by Marshall B. Rosenberg. It can be helpful in everyday communication as well as in peaceful conflict resolution in personal, professional or political areas. It does not see itself as a technique that should move other people to a certain action, but a basic attitude in which an appreciative relationship is in the foreground. Synonyms are empathetic communication, communicative communication, language of the heart, «giraffe language» (Wikipedia).

how to do something, the best way is by attacking him.

Resilience by relationships
It has been found that in no field of ability-building, the so-called primary and secondary imitation are as fully effective as in language acquisition. Primary imitation is when what is seen, is immediately imitated. Secondary imitation is when the child perceives something intensely and repeatedly, but only imitates and executes it hours or sometimes even days later.

In pedagogy, Rudolf Steiner never tires of emphasizing that in the first three years, children sensitively take into account the attitude of a person when speaking, the way he communicates. Every nuance of love and hate, the whole way of expression, the language of deeds, the way adults address and work with each other, how they shape their relationships, becomes part of the pattern adopted by children.

We know from resiliency research that for children coming from violent milieus and still developing to a certain degree in a healthy way, the so-called protective factors are affective.

What can protect a child who experiences much that is aggressive, negative? What can help him to retain in the inner core of his own being, the ability for loving and non-aggressive communication?

It was found that the strongest protective factor is a good human relationship. Such a relationship does not necessarily have to be at home through the primary caregiver, but may be provided by a caregiver in the neighborhood. This may even be the postman with whom the child runs along a ways, or a neighbor or the owner of the small shop in the village. It just has to be a human being in whose eyes the child feels «good», and accepted.

The three essential characteristics of a good relationship
There are three main characteristics, that determine a good relationship.

1. Honesty
A relationship is said to be «good» when the partners can rest assured that what the other person says is what he means. Transparency and honesty determine the relationship. This gives rise to confidence in the relationship.

2. Loving understanding for the other
Honesty can be very aggressive at times. If you unsparingly learn the truth at the wrong point in time, you feel devastated. But when you receive the truth in a good way at the right moment, in a loving process of dialogue where you feel that the other understands you, then you feel good in the relationship, accepted and taken seriously. Even if you have done a really «stupid thing» and this is clearly mirrored.

3. Respect for the autonomy of the other
This is about respecting the space of the other, about the sphere of freedom of the other. Cultivating a respectful, sensitive feeling for this personal space of the other and his limits, is the third crucial aspect. If

a relationship is governed only by honesty and understanding, without the experience of freedom and leeway, this relationship becomes a golden cage.

These three qualities – loving understanding, respect and honesty that leave the other free – are the basic qualities that protect and support the human being, but above all the little child. The resulting positive mode of communication strengthens the personality in the young children, makes them resilient, even if the child is exposed eighty percent of the day to negative, problematic, irreverent, incomprehensible and mendacious behaviors.

The brain as organ of relationships

The neurobiological correlate for this extremely sensitive interaction are the so-called mirror neurons, that have been extensively researched since their discovery by two Italian neurobiologists.

Thomas Fuchs says in his book «The Brain as an Organ of Relationship;»[2] It is the *person* who shapes the brain through their practicing, relationship-shaping behaviors on all levels.

This new view finds its crucial basis in the mirror-neuron-research. It has been demonstrated in this research that the person perceives what happens in the environment and then uses his primary and secondary imitation capacity.

Both the perception of an action and one's own, practicing, imitative activity, mirror themselves in the cortex of our brain. This is how the brain develops. In the first three years of life, the largest organization of the brain takes place and this forms the basis for later learning- and development processes.

I have already mentioned that an undisturbed and autonomy-promoting movement development is the condition for later independence and immunity against drug addiction and other addictive factors. If the acquisition of language, the development of the mode of communication on the verbal and the gestural level, is as beneficial as possible, i.e. based on a good culture of relationship, this is the strongest «remedy» against violence in later life. A person, who had to «swallow» consistently and never learned to express himself freely, to be fair and respect the space of the other, and to deal with them in a consistent manner, will behave aggressively. The reason for this is that he was already disturbed in his movement development. To understand this is a great challenge for the early childhood pedagogy.

The young child, the highest demand

Rudolf Steiner says clearly and unequivocally that the younger the children are, the higher are the moral requirements on the educators. The most glaring example was that an upper school teacher, the mathematician and physicist Ernst Lehrs, asked Rudolf Steiner if it were possible for him to lead a primary school class from one to eight in the Waldorf School in Stuttgart. Rudolf Steiner replied: «Dear Lehrs, you will have to settle for a few more years for upper school teaching». His moral matur-

---

2 Thomas Fuchs, *The brain – an organ of relationships*. Stuttgart 2010.

ity was not yet commensurate with the needs of the lower grades.

Tomorrow, when we bring together a few things about thinking, we will understand even better why that is. It is comforting that as a young educator one can replace the missing competence with love and enthusiasm. Most important is, that despite all the frustration, we do not want to let the joy of life and enthusiasm for development be spoiled.

The three phases of Communication

How does Communication come about? What processes underlie the communication process?

1. Hearing

First the perception, the hearing takes place. Through listening the inner soul realm opens. Yesterday we dealt with the outer movement realm that opens up via eye and touch. Today we will enter into the inner realm that occurs in time, and that is shaped by an inner dynamic: it is made accessible by the ear.

2. The «resonating» inside

There resonates, all that was expressed in sounds and tones, in moods, by *how* it was said and formulated, and imprints itself, when it is imitated, as a soul-neurological experience.

3. The personal statement

This leads finally to an active expression of the child. Now the child is directing, not the adult. It is special to observe a child who sees a hat lying around and says: «That is daddy!» To this the mother says lovingly «That is daddy's hat». In this way the child learns grammar: Children take over the direction of acquiring grammar by pointing to a detail and then expecting that the adults take on the sensible linguistic-grammatical ordering imbedded in context. That is why we should never speak baby talk. It is important to answer in a beautifully formulated language so that children can imitate. When we speak with one-year-olds the wonderful children's prayer by Rudolf Steiner «*From my head to my toes I am the image of God*»[3], the children begin after a while to speak along. My brother repeated the lines «in animal and flower», «in tree and stone» several times, because he liked them so much: «animal and flower, animal and flower, tree and stones, tree and stones,» When it was continued, «... nothing gives me fear», he did not speak it at all because that was scary to him. When the prayer was finished, he jumped out of bed and with the words «It is beautiful!» he threw himself down again into the pillows. This was not an expression of rational understanding but a heartfelt, emotional connection in experiencing and realizing.

Uprightness for educators

The verse that we speak here at the Goetheanum during the young-child conferences, summarizes this and can serve as an inner moral guide to uprightness for the care taking adult. Whenever we have the feeling that once again we did not

---

[3] Rudolf Steiner, *Truth Wrought Words.* GA 40.

make it, then it can be a help to deal with the truth. For upright-strength and honesty are connected: Honesty is the will to say the truth. The protective power that adults need again and again comes from the renewal of will in the contemplation of a profoundly true word configuration. Through the spirit, the relationship to God, there comes into being that which guides us through life. This is what we represent, when we offer protective forces to the children by meeting them in a loving, respectful relationship. The will for this can be strengthened by the following words by Rudolf Steiner:

«In the pure rays of light
glows the Godhead of the worlds.
In the pure love to all beings
Shines the Divinity of my soul.
I rest in the Godhead of the world.
I will find myself
in the Godhead of the world.»[4]

---

[4] Rudolf Steiner, *Meditations for the Time of Day and Seasons of the Year*, Rudolf Steiner Press, 2018. GA 267.

Birgit Krohmer
Concerning the Culture of Relationships
Examples from the practice

There is no question that we speak today of circles of devils.
Why do we not speak just as well of «circles of angels»?
Yesterday we had the five-star and the members of the human being here on the blackboard. They are connected with us we all have them. When we ask ourselves – *How can I be a role model? Have I developed myself enough? From what source can we draw?* –, we can connect with this star, let it pass through us so that the members of the human being become tuned like an instrument. There is much room for a «part» of the spiritual world – we have not been expelled from it. Angels are working on the small child. They have not left us – but we must turn to them.

I would like to point out a possibility of a tuning in to an attitude that takes less time than brushing one's teeth. You can take it up every morning in the group. You need not use this verse or do it in this way but we should find something that has this effect: *«From the head to the foot, from the heart unto my hands I am the image of God».*

I am created after the image of God. Here we are role models, we are ahead of the children. When this consciousness flows through us, we recognize a piece of heaven and not just the everyday burden that oppresses us and makes us small. *«From the head to the foot, from the heart unto the hands I am the image of God.»* Rudolf Steiner gives us here as motive: Educating means to learn to breathe. He did not mean huffing and puffing ...

When the child comes from the continuous care in the womb, s/he experiences an infinite number of polarities. The big topic that begins after birth is, being by oneself and being together. Much later come day and night. Being safe, being held, feeling well and cared for, all this is a prerequisite for the self to become active in the world in a confident way.

Speak to the child

In the language of gesture, the pleading gesture is a sign for peacefulness – in contrast to the clenched fist. We find these gestures also in words. I would like to begin with a quote from Emmi Pikler who richly rewarded us:

Even if we have the feeling that the child does not understand everything we say, or perhaps nothing we say, we will not behave as if we were mute. Let us trust that the infant can understand us when we speak naturally and simply with him.[1]

I see these words as instructions for care givers, as help for self development. We should speak to the child it does not matter whether he understands.
For how should he learn a language if he does not hear it?
I experience at work that speaking to the child has a harmonizing effect. Generally, the danger exists to say nothing, because no one asks and no one answers. But without hearing words the child does not grow into the language. On the other hand, sometimes I experience that the child is overwhelmed by language and what is said passes him by. How does this sound to

---

[1] Emmi Pikler, *Friedliche Babys – zufriedene Mütter*. Freiburg 1995. (Peaceful Babies – Content Mothers)

you: «I will get you ready quickly and then we will do this and that»? The child cannot understand everything at once. By talking while I am doing, I help myself to be present with my thoughts.

There is a language of gestures, an acting in harmony. For this we do not need words, the gestures are speaking. Above all, it is about being present and accompanying the child, to guide him with gestures, with hands, but also with words. I am in body, soul and spirit a role model for the child. The younger the children are the more they look right through us. They are not yet imitating us adults after we have done something, they imitate us during our doing.

Imitating the present – Imitating the past

I ask parents often if they can remember how it was when they wanted to go out for the first time without their child. The following answer is exemplary: «We started very early to remain calm but our child was very active. We took an extra long walk with him to get him tired in the fresh air». The child was so awake because the parents were excited, and the child imitated the mood – «Today we have a lot going». In that case we can say good bye with these words: «I will be back». We are deeply connected with the children via our human organizational members.

It is soothing, to attune our various members so that they become ordered. I will now show a brief movie that deals with sensitivity in the finger tips and about gestures that announce a peaceful intention: the child is at an age, when he could not have been taught anything yet. The child, who would like to have a small cloth stops briefly before he takes the cloth, and asks for it. This is pure imitation, because this was always done by others around him.

We find soul-spiritual qualities such as «honesty» and the ability to have a point of view, also in the physical. The word «fingertip feeling» is rarely used for a fine motor ability. But there it has its origin. Relationship arises in the now, in the encounter. Every moment is unique.

However, if we take such pictures with us as an expectation of ourselves, or as requirement of the children, then we fall out of the here and now. Then we are only in the head.

Hands and gestures

Hands are ambassadors and scouts. They perceive much during care-taking, and they can say much. The one hand touches the child, so that the thumb is removed from the mouth. The other points to the shoulder, where the care taker would like to tie the sleeping bag: «I want to button your sleeping bag, will you take that little thumb out of your mouth?» Whether that is said in words or not is not that important. The key is that we understand each other. That we communicate – with gestures, with looks, with words. Angela understood, otherwise she would not smile. If these two would not lead a «together-dialogue», they would have an «against each other-dialogue» that would also be possible. A child who is used to having his thumb pulled out of his mouth, reacts differently. The together, or the against-each-other starts early, still on the tonus-level after birth. It grows also, we do not notice it for a long time.

Here I will show another sequence, «acting in harmony». This is not yet done in formal terms the child is not yet meaningfully active. But s/he imitates the gesture language, the finger-agility, the skillfulness that he perceives during the care-taking. I like to speak about imitating as the «together with» (mitahmen) of the young child. He enters directly into our intention and our doing. We see what a pleasure it can be to be taken care of.

Dialogue in doing

We see an orphan with a care-taker during her shift. Angela takes off her little stockings. These are moments in which one senses how the temporal process is shaped. Only the adult is responsible for this. The nurse waits to see if Angela likes to adjust the sock a bit more, if the child pushes it to the heel, so she can take it. What is important is that this is a joint activity, where you share hand movements and enter into a dialogue, where the child feels perceived.

Creating a real dialogue during care-taking not only helps to satisfy the child's needs, but it is also an important social experience for the child. An infant who is more or less participating in common activity, experiences that his signals were noticed and well understood. The fact that his activity is accepted during feeding, dressing and undressing, gives him the feeling that he can influence the situation in which he is involved. This trust is a good basis for his first social relationships.[2]

The ability to communicate is often stifled even before the language is added as body-free communication, because we do not know that we *always* communicate, and therefore do not respond to each other in an answering and questioning way. By that I do not mean that we should ask the children: «Do you want tea, juice, banana or cookie?» To ask these questions is a time sickness. It is about making a deep communicative connection when learning to walk, to speak, and to think: I first understand the gesture language, the language of movement. Later I understand the words and in the activity I understand the meaning.

The acquisition of speech a gift from Heaven

If we treat the children with care, we can look «into heaven» during the language acquisition period. Because the angels are still working on them, we can look through the children and experience other spheres. That gives us strength. When children begin to use words, these are often more exact then those of the adults – that is, if we listen well to them and do not immediately correct.

I would like to give a few examples: A child reaches with his hand for a mug and says: «The tea must first warm off.» Do

---

[2] Ute Strub, Anna Tardos (Hg.), *Im Dialog mit dem Säugling und Kleinkind*. Pikler Gesellschaft Berlin 2006. (in conversation with infants and small children)

you feel that it has to «cool off», when it is still too hot? The formulation – «The tea must warm off» – is more exact, and corresponds much more to the process.

Or: «My doll is in love. Especially in the face and on the hands». It is wonderful to listen to children and notice that their use of language is more exact than ours. With their thoroughness they present us with rich gifts.

Develop joy in discovery

I often get calls from parents who want advice because their child does not seem to be developing. As a rule, only those parents ask for an educational consultation who try hard, are thorough and also worried. When I have the impression that the child is healthy – if s/he were not healthy, he would need a pediatrician more than an education councilor – I advise parents to buy a nice little book. They will have an appointment earliest in four weeks, and they get the task to write into the booklet what discovery they make each day. As a rule, I could spend my first counseling session by listening to all that is not yet functioning. That does not interest me. I encourage the parents to write every day what they discovered about their child, even some small change. For, it just cannot be that a child does not develop:

Does the child open and close his hand?
Does the hand find the mouth?
Does he sleep for 24 hours?

Naturally not! I experience that most parents say after two to three weeks: «It is already much better». After three to four weeks they say: «At the moment I do not need the appointment. I will call back in four weeks».

The educational atmosphere – to use a professional term – and the relationships have changed because these parents are no longer looking into the cradle, with the question of what their child lacks, but with the will to discover something. While I discover, encounters take place. The discovering gaze of the adult, attending to the development of the child and perceiving what he is working on at the moment, is like the sun for the flower. The moment a connection happens both learn to support one another and to do well with one another. That is why I warned at the beginning to derive a standard from the pictures. Every example, every spiritual direction, every statement runs the risk of becoming a dogma. There are some parents who come to the admittance interview and say, «unfortunately, my child spoke before he walked.» Then I ask: «Was he still lying on his back?» – «No! of course not». He has already gone through a good deal of movement development, otherwise he could not have begun to speak. As a rule, development is coherent if we don't think in terms of «Milestones» and «stops», but understand it as process. Like the tea that still has to «warm down». As soon as we understand ourselves to be in such a procedural connection, there arises a common process that is shaped together.

Tuning in to one another in dialogue

I have been working on a book lately and have repeatedly been asked: «Write a few nice dialogues, so that we can read, how to talk to children. Many cannot do that anymore today». But I could not write any dialogues. I have many in my ear that I heard from myself as a mother and from others. The moment we are dealing with other people, the dialogues must change, must become dialogues between these particular people. Only that way would they be consistent.

We have an incredible sense for voice, mood, tone and sound. One can say: «Will you please give me your *hand*?», or «*Will you please* give *me your hand*?» Do you hear the difference? We don't do this with a child! The mother tongue is how I carry the language in me, and how it comes out. Then it is consistent.

I believe, we cannot write any dialogues for other people because talks are intimate meetings, intimate encounters. In an encounter, the I of the one who is active, reveals itself. If the care-giving is good, then both are active. However, the *how* is totally individual. Gaining uprightness is an act of the most intimate self-assertiveness. Out of the language, the inner being sounds forth. If we use a dialogue according to a text book, it becomes automatic. Then we no longer listen to the children.

Little children are unbelievably pure mirrors. They are not yet pretending. They reflect us as no one else in the world could do it. This is our greatest help for self-education – provided we enjoy looking in that mirror.

Michaela Glöckler
Awakening in the environment

Our conference has three main themes: The first two, the principle of autonomy and the cultural principle of development, were the topics of the last days. The latter implies that all development takes place in encounters and only through encounters. Without encounter, there is no development. Development is a creative process of the space between beings and things (subject and object) – that is why education, if it wants to promote development, is the forming of relational spaces.

The riddle of the development of self-consciousness

The third focus that will occupy us today is the awakening in the world, the mystery of consciousness. Master Ekkehard put it this way: «*If I were a king and did not know it, I would not be a king*».

If I were a wonderful, God created, incarnating human-I and did not know it, if I had no consciousness of this I, what would I be?

The significant third step is the riddle of the development of self-consciousness.

How can education help that the human being who is awakening to this self-consciousness, can have joy in it? How can it be achieved that this self-confidence grows throughout the whole biography with all the self-experience of joy and sorrow, and is not so offended when we doubt ourselves persistently, even become desperate?

This questioning makes us aware of the great drama of development.

Which being does the child call «I»?

Yesterday we saw excerpts in videos and in photos, how autonomy can be acquired. We have seen excerpts of certain activities that have been carried out with concentrated attention. The gaze, the grasp and the object formed a self-contained moving wholeness that was closely related to the sum of all activities that the child experiences from morning to evening. This includes being fed regularly, cared for – all accompanied by the loving gazes of adults, by an environment that carries. The child experiences the etheric touch in the gaze of the educator: She only has to look at him briefly, and immediately the child is reconnected with the wholeness of the environment, to the sum of the activities, that he himself accomplished and experienced.

I am all this

The child learns by imitating a role model or s/he is encouraged «to imitate together with», to actively participate. Creating opportunities for this in the child's environment is the task of the educators. When the child says «I» to himself in the third year of life, he then summarizes a body and soul- psycho-social, object-related wholeness. Everything that the child related himself to awaken his self, complemented it, opened it. To all that was remembered, to all the actions that he co-performed, to the many small exercised processes in autonomous self-activity, to all this the child says in the end: «I am all this. But now nothing will happen anymore without my self-consciousness!»

We can all remember our first ego experience. From that time on, our self-consciousness, our «I- thought», accompanies us throughout our life. Our I- consciousness accompanies our biography and is part of everything. Everything is being watched! We constantly watch ourselves, as the care giver watched us. In the retrospect every evening, we can reinforce this by letting our day pass in review and saying to ourselves: All this was you!

Where am I, when I speak of myself in terms of «you»?

It is an elementary experience to realize clearly that our consciousness, our thinking, is based on an out-of-body experience. Out-of-body experience! In thinking, in our reflective self-awareness, we are active out-of-body, and therefore we can place everything before us, can see ourselves from the outside. Hölderlin put it this way: «*Those who step on their misery, stand higher*». He found that he could go through the worst hell, but that he was not hell himself. He could look at hell.

Do you understand the difference? I am not identical with the moment of life in which I am currently active, in which, by virtue of my individual body and soul structure, I am «stuck», by virtue of my incarnation. I'm not just that, I'm also the one who looks at everything and therefore also stands elsewhere!

Consciousness of our humanity

Anthroposophy is a Greek word and means: «Knowledge or wisdom of man». Rudolf Steiner translated it for himself: «Anthroposophy is consciousness of my humanity, my humanness». We can ask ourselves every day:

How far has the consciousness of my humanity, my humanness matured?

Every human being can ask himself that, whether he knows Anthroposophy or not. When we think back, we can bring before us, how we were five years ago, how ten years ago – and we can imagine how it will be in ten years. When we know – this is what I want to learn! – we are in the mood full of expectation, like a child when he says to himself «I» and suddenly notices: I am here, I am conscious of myself, I want something.

The awakening of self-consciousness happens by experiencing and confronting the world. The child summarizes his relation to the world in this «I am».

The thought: I am I

A person who later became a physicist and a psychiatrist, had his first I-experience in Israel at the beach of Haifa. He stood there as little boy and saw at the horizon something like a little stick stretching straight up. This little stick came closer and closer, became bigger. He saw a second little stick emerging behind. This shape lifted further and further out of the sea and became a ship with a mast and sails. The boy stood and watched how this ship pulled into the harbor at Haifa. His first personal thought as consequence of this experience was: The earth must be round! He had played often with a ball and observed, how the printed patterns appear one after the other, when one rolls a ball from the back to the front. From this example it becomes clear, that saying I is connected with a first conscious thought achievement. This «I am I» experience can be remembered in form of a picture or can materialize in a situation, where we would ask: Why is this like that? We often remember what thought came to us in connection with the experience: «I am I».

The essence of Life
Rudolf Steiner's new paradigm in education and medicine is based on groundbreaking research results all around the essence of the living, i.e. the etheric. He spoke of two fundamental things in connection with this wonderful world of life.

When the chemist Rudolf Hauschka asked him, «Tell me, doctor, what is life?», Rudolf Steiner answered: «Study the rhythms! Rhythm bears life!» It is clear then, that lack of rhythm puts children under stress, makes them insecure and damages them in their life sphere with the result of illness.

The second fundamental realization was the discovery of the fact that the material that thoughts are made off is pure life, that the life in our body is identical in essence with our thought life. We grow in our thoughts, we develop spiritually with the help of the same etheric forming forces that the body uses to grow and develop itself. Rudolf Steiner said to the doctors:

«It is of the greatest importance to know, that the normal thought-forces of the human are the transformed growth and -regeneration forces.»[1]

With «transforming» he means the special moment, when the life- and growth forces, that the body does not need anymore, become body-free and reflect the out- of- body thought competence in the brain. These connections throw light onto the mystery of incarnation – they provide the necessary spiritual and physiological substantiation.

Speech and movement
There is something really great about language acquisition: The same intelligence inherent in language was already evident in the holistic, concerted, concentrated movements that the child had previously practiced. This has been extensively studied by language research. As a rule, it takes about three months, a trimester for the wisdom that lies in a gesture to be translated into language by the child.

How far we are today from implementing this knowledge I have recently experienced in a train. There, next to me in the large compartment sat a mother, a father and a barely two-year-old child. They had a big book with pictures in front of them. The parents showed the child individual pictures and communicated the concepts to him. The child wanted to please his parents – this was noticeable in his effort to carry on with the naming, until exhausted, he put his head on the table and went to sleep. He was then permitted to sleep for a while but when he woke up the whole thing started anew. We are dealing here with promoting the intelligence according

---

1 Rudolf Steiner, Ita Wegman, *Fundamentals of Therapy*. GA 27, Chapter 1.

to a certain program. Generation after generation is ruined by such games. This is intellectual use of force, intellectual power abuse. We speak today of verbal and body abuse.

We do not speak about such intellectual infringements. However, they are just as harmful and traumatizing as abuse of body and soul. They are a spiritual martyrdom. We have to become sensitive to this.

The decisive step is, that we bring to our consciousness the out-of-body experience-quality of our thinking. Then we will have a similar «Aha»-experience as we had on our first morning, when we discovered together the etheric realm in which mother and child are present when they look into each other's eyes – or the care person and the child or father and child. It is always about the thought realm, the realm of meaningfulness, the realm of wisdom.

Through the active role modeling of the mother or educator, and the activity of the child slowly a metamorphosis takes place, from deed, from activity, to communication via language. As you can see, the child is now able to express himself, not only intelligently in body language as in the first year, but also «air-linguistically». Speech goes out of the physical body through the air into the surrounding space, it frees itself. Every word is an out- of- body reality, speaking is an out- of- body activity. It's like a small birth for the child: he says a word and his surroundings understand it more or less well. One has to struggle to hand the words over of the air, that they reach out to the listener, as if from outside, out- of- body, as out-of-body messages, that then are internalized. The listener picks up what he hears via the body-free etheric that is in the ear. In all senses, our etheric is mobile, and loose. It can emerge and can let us perceive. The etheric body is a whole that protrudes from the sense organs and in this way comes into contact with the environment, the «sense» world. Deeply unconscious, intuitive, the sense is experienced, the sense of life.

The connection of ether body and astral body

I have to go back a bit to show that when the child learns to speak, the etheric connects with another human member, the astral body. The etheric body shapes the physical body according to the laws of the sense organs. This means, that every perception, every impression reactively also forms the body. In the course of the language forming, of language development, the etheric and astral are moved out of the body and given over to the air as a pure air formation, as an «air birth».

The second metamorphosis manifests itself in the fact, that the etheric body not only shapes the physical body in accordance with the laws of the sense organs, that it not only shapes it according to the sound forms and the tones when speaking, but that it transforms gestures into speech. This is done with the help of feeling. The astral body gives us the ability to feel. The etheric body gives us the ability to live and to think. Because of this, in many ancient spiritual systems, the etheric is shown either as a germ or in the form of an open lemniscate because it is in the essence of the etheric that one part incarnates and the other excarnates.

The etheric body is the bearer of life and thought. The astral body, on the other hand, is the bearer of feeling. Speech springs from the feeling, the longing to communicate, to speak out and to get to know the other. Yearning for communication underlies the feeling life. We want to get together, come harmoniously together. We suffer when there is disharmony, want to overcome it. For this we need speech.

I-conscious thinking

The result of the third metamorphosis is that the ego-organization is emancipated and thus body-free, I-conscious intentional thinking becomes possible. The ego-organization is the bearer of our will, of our innermost will to live.

Recently, many magazines discussed the book by Charles Fernyhough's, *The Child in the Mirror*[2]. For early childhood educators, it is worth while reading because in it a psychologist studies his daughter very carefully between the age of zero to three. He writes down every essential experience in the process of the maturing identity. When I read it, it once again opened my eyes to the essence of the etheric.

We know from Anthroposophy that underlying the whole movement development works and comes to expression the same wisdom, the same intelligence. It expresses itself in speech and in thought. It cannot be said that this wisdom would

---

[2] Charles Fernyhough, *Das Kind im Spiegel*. München 2010 (The Child in the Mirror)

only begin to work at the age of three, when the child says «I» to himself. On the contrary, the child says «I» to this wise authority who ruled over the entire development from embryonic development through birth to the moment of expressing the I. At this moment, however, he experiences himself for the first time in his ego-organization as an out-of-body and abstractly thinking being, as a self-thinking being.

Thought forces of the etheric

The etheric body models the nervous system, which in the first three years experiences the greatest neuron growth in the entire development. A three-year-old child has more neurons than a college student at prime age. The portion of neurons, which is not holistically taken hold of, seized, captured, used, will regress later. But whatever is built up in the process of neural interconnecting, will be realized individually in a large design, within the framework of what the child may learn. This etheric forming force that underlies this amazing brain formation becomes body free and thus available for the spiritual, thought-conscious life.

> But where do these etheric – and following that the astral and ego/I -forces – become body-free?
> Where is the birth place?

The location of the birth can only be in one place – the heart: the etheric body invigorates the blood by letting it flow. However, at the end of the diastole, in the diastasis, the blood content comes to a standstill for a fractions of a second. Then the next contraction of the ventricles takes place, the blood is ejected again into the body cycle and everything is brought back into circulation and moves again.

In the brief moment of the stoppage of the blood, that is only possible in the heart, those etheric forces become body-free that the body does not use anymore for the incarnation and the health maintenance. With every heart beat a small «dying and becoming» takes place. That which is not needed anymore for the self healing of the body is now needed for the spiritual healing. Spiritual healing means, to become thought- spiritually a harmonious whole, to work to understand the world, to work with love, to find oneself in the world, to bring to consciousness and become clear even about small incidents, and not to shrink back from even a most difficult destiny, but to use it to wake up.

The redeeming power of thought

In a deeply Christian fairy tale is shown how, based on an unlucky destiny a human being can repay evil with good, and it is shown, how through this action the whole culture changes. Evil should not be pursued with hatred, but should be requited with good. When Rudolf Steiner was asked why evil is in the world, he said: «*Not so that we give in to it, but that we awaken on it for the good.*»

Whenever we complain about evil in the world our will drives us to sleep. We do not want to awaken. That is why evil continues. We do not want to make an effort spiritually, in thought. We could see in the financial crisis how everything continued on in the old thought patterns. The courage to step out into a spiritual new land is not there – to step back and look what has happened in the last 200 years of the history of finance, and whether we want to continue in this way. The root of evil is the refusal to develop spiritually.

To the question on a questionnaire – *which mistake would you most readily forgive?* – the young Rudolf Steiner answered: *Each one as soon as I understand it.*

That is ingenious! I can forgive every mistake as soon as I understand it. That is the redeeming, healing power of thinking, this wonderful, free force of thinking, given into the hands of the human-I, the pure body-free force of thinking that is not bound to body nor soul dependency. With the help of this free thinking ability we can penetrate, re-work, order, enliven everything that surrounds us, but also are able to dispose of whatever is necessary.

Self-awakening in thinking

A child succeeds in the powerful self-awakening in thinking, if he was allowed to experience this intelligent competence already in the development of movement, in autonomous activity of his own accord. If there was a space in which he was allowed to hear and speak, in which he could reflect and become aware of himself, in which he could learn to find his own words, to form his own sentences, without being constantly corrected, if he was allowed to unfold without having to imitate baby talk. It's not about expressions like «tucki, tucki», but about false words that are offensive to the etheric. If this process of self-awakening was possible, the mind of the person in question will be strong, self-confident and creative, and able to bring something new into the world, that will transform the world.

Claudia Grah-Wittich
Awakening in the environment: Examples from the practice

> «Create for yourself moments of inner peace and in these moments
> learn to distinguish the essential from the nonessential.»[1]
> Rudolf Steiner

When we talk about the environment of the young child, I want to differentiate between the external environment and the inner environment. In the outer world, we are all professionals and specialists. All over the world, where I have seen institutions in the spirit of Waldorf education, they are aesthetically beautiful. In recent years, however, the child's inner environment has become more and more important to me: And this is all of us, the adults – that's why I call us the child's first environment. I would like to activate the same aesthetics, the same harmony, in the adults. Instead of «inner environment» I want to choose the concept of «space».

Experiment to care for the inner space

I will do a little exercise with you now. The experiment will take five to six minutes. You are allowed to talk briefly with your neighbor, about what you have heard or what is important to you.

Step 1 of the Exercise: Have a brief conversation with each other.

Step 2: Create this inner peace for a moment. Go into contemplation, look inward, stay with yourself. Sort a little bit:

> Where do you stand right now?
> How are you?
> Are you in yourself?

---

[1] Rudolf Steiner, *Wie erlangt man Erkenntnisse der höheren Welten?* GA 10, p. 22.

> Are you here or already on your trip home?

Look inside and see what goes on in you, what thoughts and feelings do you have. A moment of inner peace.

Step 3: Continue the conversation with your neighbor.

I will tell you now how I utilize this exercise in the seminars, and I hope that this also meets your experience. The conversation of the third step went perhaps this way, that you heard more, listened more, paid more attention and you did not have so much the intention to communicate something. Evaluate your experiences briefly, and if I am lucky, you were able to recognize the difference in quality of the short conversation, and what it means to look even one minute into yourself. If the experiment worked, you can take this experience along, if it did not it would be worth trying it again!

The hygienic principle in pedagogy

For me the secret of pedagogy is this: Do not get bogged down. That I am not driven to go where I don't want to, but practice consequently to take this moment of inner peace and focus on soul hygiene, look inward:

> Where do I stand right now?
> What do I feel?
> What is my intention?
> Am I present?
> Did life drive me somewhere where I do not want to be?
> Am I master of the house?

In this presence you can perceive children more delicately, because you are present in

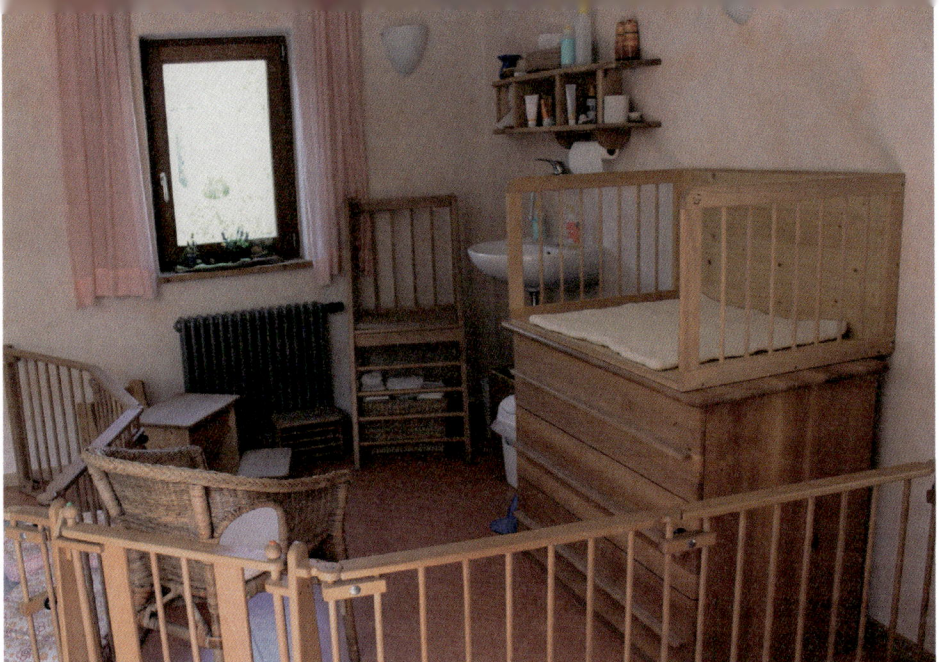

Fig. 1

yourself. You will notice that you do not get as tired as when you occupy yourself otherwise. I will be glad when this becomes your wish. A paradigm change will occur in education when we understand ourselves as space, and begin to see the care of the inner space as an important hygienic principle. We should provide quiet for ourselves – before each teachers' meeting, before each moment when we are in front of the children, and always when we feel that we lose ourselves, and go where we do not want to go. We must learn to see ourselves as first environment of the child. This is especially the case with the young child who looks directly and deeply into us.

Let us experiment and come into an exchange concerning the creation of moments of inner peace. Let us practice this in the meetings, seminars, and in further education! This seems to me more important than to speak about how we create outer spaces. The latter will happen when we discover the beauty, harmony and rhythm of our inner space.

I wanted to conclude by expressing my respect for Emmi Pikler with this thought that I regard myself as the first environment of the child, and I will bring two pictures. When I experience mindfulness, respect, reverence and love for the child and treat him accordingly, then the child can take this experience through imitation and transform it in play. This, in turn can then become an inner attitude that he takes out into the world. The pedagogy of Emmi Pikler is a peace pedagogy, when we notice how peaceably and mindful interactions take place.

Shaping the outer space

The outer space must be structured in such a way that it can give orientation to the child. The aesthetics result from clearly articulated functions, that we also find in ourselves. The clear structure of the room is necessary for the children, so that they may know what will happen where and when. What is happening when, where, with whom, for what? This must

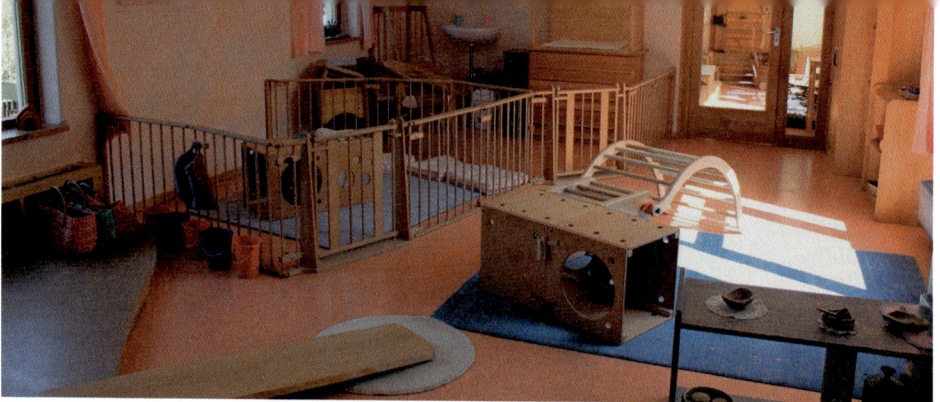

Fig. 2

always be your question when you arrange and set up the rooms.

– The care takers realm

There must be a place where the children are cared for – the care area (Pflegebereich). The child needs to know that there is someone in this area, a care taker, who can support him on his way to become self-sufficient.

In the «Wiegestube» at the «hof» this area is bordered so that no other children can pull on the skirt of the care-taker and make her lose concentration. Nevertheless, there are other children playing in the room. Should a child in the playroom need the attention of the care person, she will turn to the playing children briefly. Care-taking does not need to happen in a closed off room. This can serve as a model: When children can observe and perceive how diapers are put on and taken off in one area, and how in another area they will get something to eat, we can observe that also in the play activity of the children, we find that quality of quiet and deep concentration. Here we are active as role models for the children in a necessary and meaningful activity.

There must be a clearly defined care area that is well secured. The children should have complete autonomy, even when they are cared for with diaper changing, and being dressed and undressed. They may choose to stand up when diapers are changed, which is possible because they can hold on, or choose to lie down. Often children shift positions during a diaper change. Changing diapers while standing does not take longer, than when lying down. There is also a table where older children can climb up and stand.

– Play-area

Here is the play area. There are several things where children can climb up. There is an area for younger children so that they are not disturbed by the older ones when they play and jump around. The younger ones have another possibility to play in a protected area but still they are part of everything – also in the protected space where they can develop.

How we design all this in detail depends really on the situation of the overall space. In the play-room is an area with closets that have a curtain. One of the nicest games for children is called: «Cuckoo»: close the curtain, open the curtain, I am gone, now I am back. A primal experience, an archetypal game for each child.

I would like to address the forming of the inner space again:
Where am I now?
What am I doing?

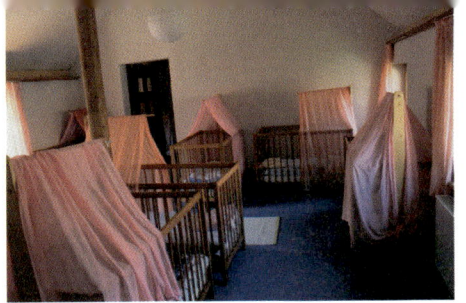

Fig. 3

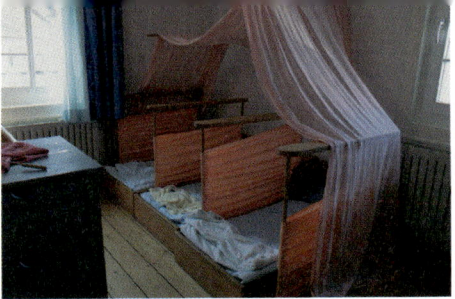

Fig. 4

When am I doing it?
How do I form it and for what?

An educator accompanies a child while getting her dressed after the nap. She has a safe position, she is sitting comfortably. An important message that I want to express clearly is: Make sure that you feel well. When you take good care of yourself then you can also care well for others. You do not need to struggle so much, feel stressed and then carry the stress outside – to the parents and into the meetings. Try to do your work in a way that corresponds with the task but also corresponds with yourself. Sit down when you attend to a child who dresses him/herself. In the coatroom, you can sit down – if you do not take along too many children and then have to jump from one to another. It's a good idea to dress children one after the other as long as they still need help. This guarantees the child their full attention and at the same time he can do a much by himself. Observe the variety of movement that takes place during such a dressing process, when the sweater is not simply slipped over, but the arm slips into the jacket:

What does the child examine what does he learn about his own body?
What bodily activities are taking place?
What is his concentration, what intensity is displayed?
Where does the foot reappear from the pant-leg?

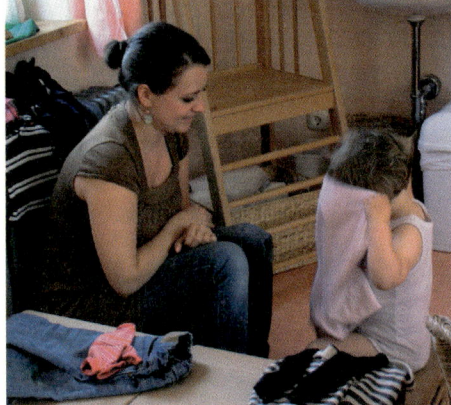

Fig. 5

We need to find a suitable space for dressing.

– The Eating area

As a mother, I am very familiar with what I later learned in Pikler-pedagogy. When a child is weaned, it goes without saying that we take him into our personal space and feed him on our lap.

I sit down comfortably, take, for example a stool to put my feet on. If I feel safe, then the child can also feel safe and concentrate well on the process of eating. That is not easy, much has to be coordinated: chewing, swallowing, taking the spoon between the lips. It is a learning process: Wait till the mouth is empty, wait till it is opened again. We have to be in contact with the child during this process. We succeed best when we are inwardly calm.

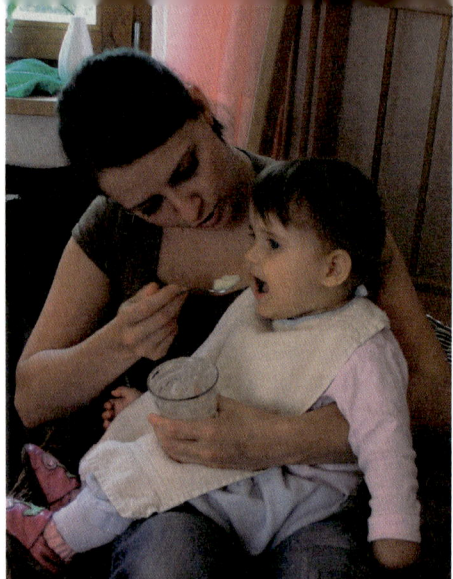

Fig. 6

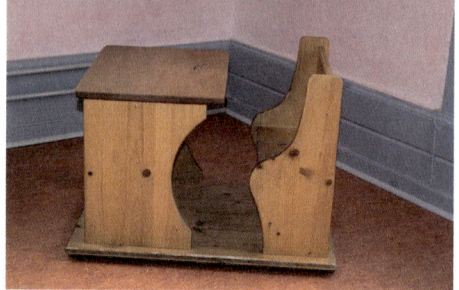

Fig. 7

As a mother, I did not eat at the table with all children right away when they were still little. When a child was no longer sitting on my lap, I sat down beside him at the table, attended to him and waited until he could take the spoon himself and could coordinate between taking it, laying down it again, and estimating how much he should take. When a child could do that, he had found his way into the family.

Eating benches make sense because a child can be attended to during the process of learning this cultural ability. This process takes a certain amount of time, but you should not set a time, how long it should be. Children who already eat independently sit in small groups at low tables. Here giving and taking can begin as a first social process. This can only take place when the basic skills are mastered. Eating with many small children in a group is unlikely to be a social event when everyone is busy wiping food stains, spilled glasses.

If you want to design physical spaces out of your inner space, you should ask yourself:

How do I create the necessary peace, so that children can enter into the learning processes?

Education is self-education

These were examples for the creation of outer spaces with the consciousness of the inner space. The appropriate designing of the surroundings of the child is a prerequisite for communication, relationship skills, and autonomy to develop on their own. As a human being who educates herself, I have to enter the process, and should not look at education as something I do for the children – I have to consider myself as learner of the child. The following quote by Rudolf Steiner about self-education is important to me. In view of this we could organize a congress with the theme: «Self-education».

This education is self-education. Actually, as teachers and educators, we are only the environment of the child who is educating himself. We have to be the best environment, so that the child can educate himself, as it must according to his inner destiny.[2]

This concludes the series of topics ranging from autonomy via the relationship culture to structuring the environment.

---

[2] Rudolf Steiner, *The Child's Changing Consciousness and Waldorf Education*. GA 306, Eight lectures, Dornach, 15. to 22. April 1923. Sixth lecture, 20. April 1923.

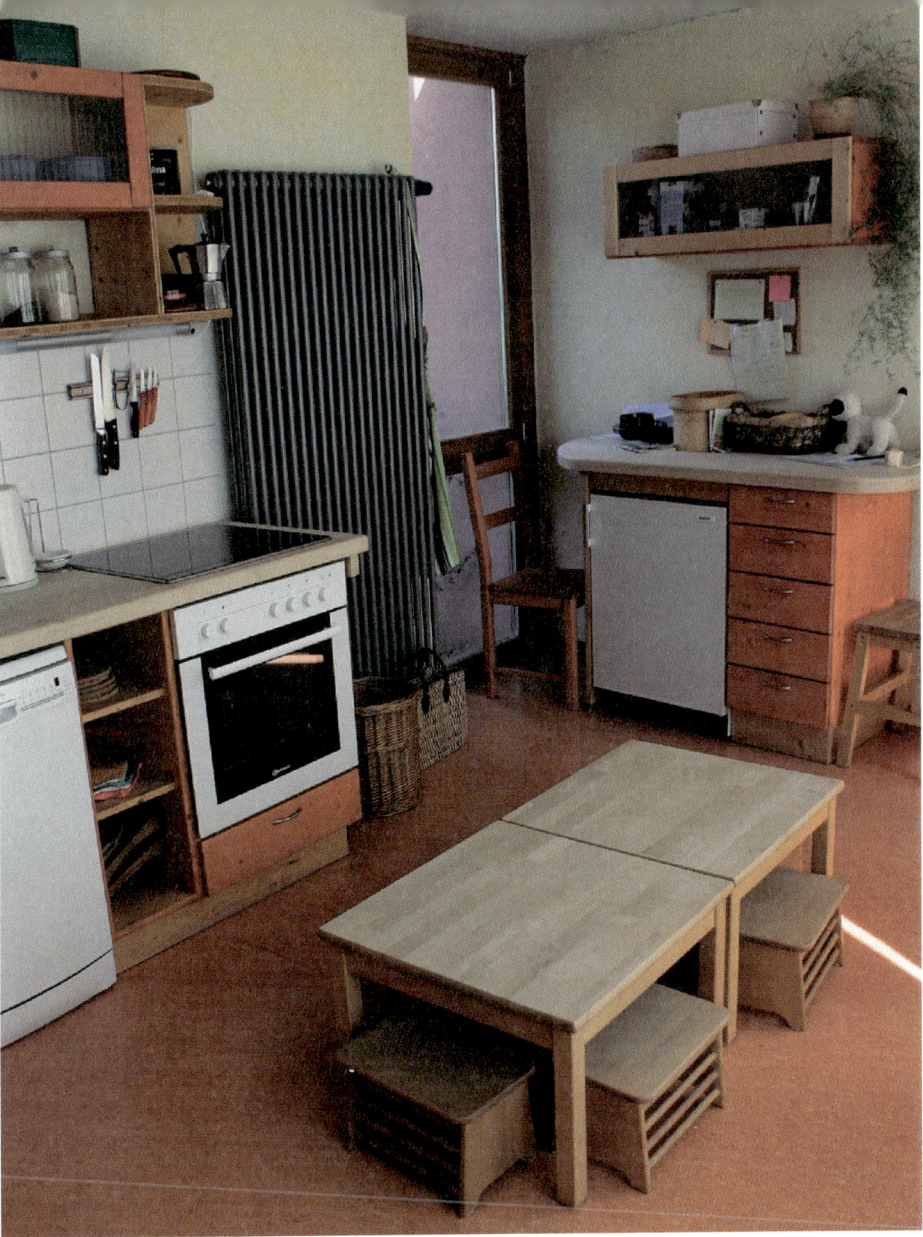

Fig. 8

Claudia Grah-Wittich
An Example from the Practice

In every perception lives a discovery. I would like to show you a short sequence, where we can notice that observation can be the path to our own freedom. We can only bring children to freedom, when we know our own freedom, when we enjoy it and know how to handle it. Freedom has much to do with warmth and at the same time with refreshment.

When you get tired in the everyday practice, feel totally stuck in your work, and would prefer to go home, try to look at the children again – try to perceive them. You will find that you are refreshed when you discover something new in the children. The tiredness leaves you, joy rises up, and warmth fills you. The child and you are in a dialogue that initially has nothing to do with speaking.

Emilio

I want to show you a scene with Emilio, who is jumping off a set of play-stairs for the first time. I ask you to look at the scene without bias. Afterwards, we will look at a section posing a particular question.

First, I want to bring a comparison: Imagine, a mother says to her schoolchild: «It is time to do your homework! Settle down!» She wants her child to stay focused. The groundwork necessary to develop the ability to stay on task needs to be laid in a young child already, by giving him space and not interrupting him.

In this film you can see Emilio's concentration. It was a coincidence that he discovered that you can jump off. He was surprised at his own doing. He repeats the jump again and again – he practices! Then comes the moment when he seems tired. Nevertheless, he still continues.

I want you to pay attention to how Emilio lands on the floor: on the first jump he was tired after climbing the stairs. Nevertheless, he jumped again. For what reason? What motivated him?

- He falls on his stomach and then turns on his back. Like a baby, with his arms and hands up, he rolls on his back for a while. From the safety of this baby position, he gets up again and jumps.
- He lands sideways now, then gets down on his knees and crawls.
- Next time he lands in the quadruped stand.
- Finally he lands upright.

Up to this point, the entire movement development from lying on the floor to uprightness is gone through again. Amazing body knowledge! Emilio first needed the safety of lying on the floor in order to integrate the new experience (jumping down), then to switch to creeping and crawling and finally to standing up. No one showed it to him, no one advised him! He knew that in order to continue practicing, he needed to gain self-confidence from those earlier positions in his movement development.

From each level, however, he goes into the upright again – isn't that wonderful? We can look at this as a conquest of the consciousness of freedom.

With regard to this film sequence we have to ask ourselves:

How much time do children have on the stairs?
How many children get this time to enjoy their movements in peace?

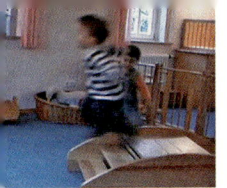 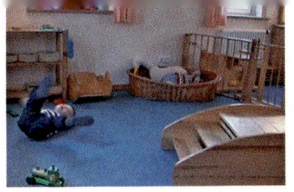 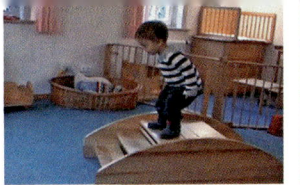 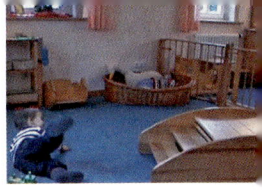
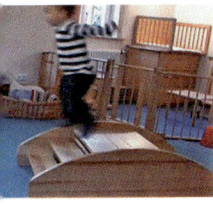 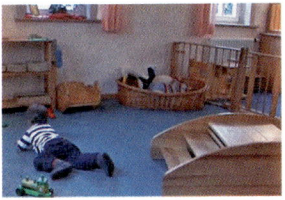 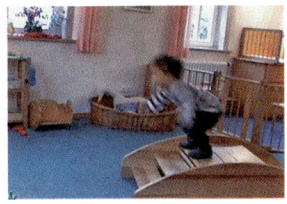 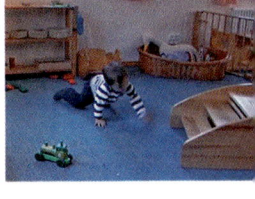
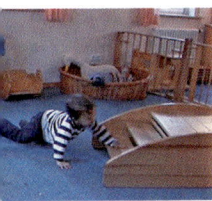 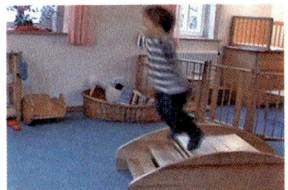 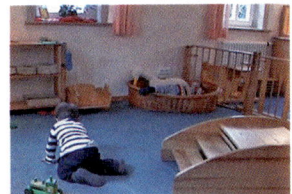 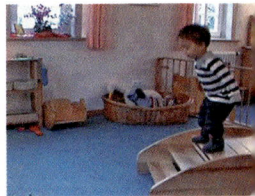
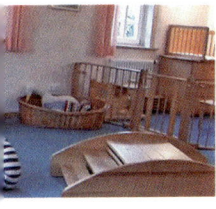 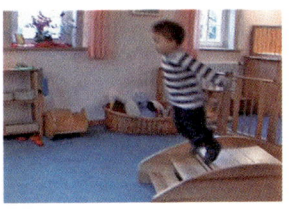 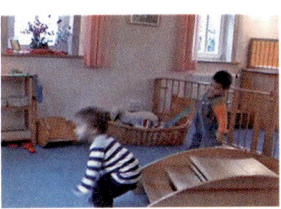 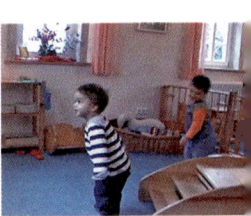

How much of their time do children spend on the move, because they are taken somewhere?

The example shown should serve as a suggestion for your own discoveries. The prerequisite is that you give the children time. In Emilio's case, nobody was annoyed because he jumped again and again and took up space in the group.

Try to discover what children do out of their deep body knowledge to feel secure in such a thing like the jump! Become an explorer – in the interest of children and in your own!

Birgit Krohmer
Educational quality through documentation

I would like to invite you into a workshop and put forward some thoughts, which I hope will also underlie the research and work of many of you.

I got to know Emmi Pikler in 1980. For me it was a destiny meeting. Two years later, now 28 years ago, I was writing my dissertation at the Waldorf-Education-Seminar. The topic was a compilation of what could be found in Rudolf Steiner and in Emmi Pikler about the first three years of life. There were no keywords at that time – it was a relative new territory.

Help to save childhood

We can find infinitely many treasures in both movements. In many areas they even correspond. I would like to compare and connect several aspects. The order is not meant to be a value judgment. If you have occupied yourself for many years with a topic, it starts on its own to connect itself and become one. For me, it is no longer so important to ask where my knowledge comes from, but how it gets to the child. I would like to encourage all of us, to learn to rediscover childhood as a space for development, and put it into words. We should try to bring the subject of «childhood» close to every person in a society, so that childhood can take its proper place in the long term, no matter what our relationship to the child may be. Every moment in childhood that can be saved is precious.

Concerning development much is measured and standardized today. Many parents are asking nervously whether their child is «normal» and developing in a healthy way. It is not enough anymore to say to them: «He will be fine, give him time!» This does not reassure them. It is also not about calming their fears but to encourage them to change their perspective so that they can learn to discover the child's development and be able to enjoy it. The more we know the laws of development, the more we can discover in the children.

The three-steps of development

I start with a shape you probably already know – the three-step. According to the *Theosophy*, we could assign: 21 years, 42 years, 63 years – the developmental periods of the body members, the soul- and the spirit members.

Each of them can be divided into three seven-year cycles. Our grandparents would have assigned the first seven years to be at home, the second seven years to the elementary school time and the third to apprenticeship and the traveling-years.

Rudolf Steiner divided this three-step of the seven-year cycles further according to the laws of the body corporeality into head, trunk and limbs:
- Half-round and closed off (head) – the activity is directed to the inside
- straight, like rays, turned to the outside (limbs) – the activity is directed to the outside world
- flexible middle (trunk) mediates between the two poles and directions.

Steiner described, how these areas can be further divided by three: The upper head, for instance, is closed, the middle part of the head is interrupted by sense organs, the lower head has a movable part (lower jaw).

When we take hold of our body and of our human members, we take this path: The head is always first in a healthy birth. It is also the first thing where the personal will of the child becomes visible, when s/he moves his little head towards us and away again. Head, trunk, limbs.

The three-step in play during the first seven years

I am giving an example of how development can be seen in three steps during the play activity of the young child:
1. In the first third of the first seven-year cycle, the child lives totally in perception. He takes everything in that he sees in the world. His playing is an experimental play all possibilities are checked out. In this way he takes hold of his body, builds his corporeality, gets to know the space, moves in space, and begins to create in space.
2. In the next third we speak of the fantasy-age.
3. In the last third, we see the play change to «I would» and «you could» and «then we would» – the role- play. Here planning takes place and a will-intention is set.

Such three-steps we find in a refined way again and again.

The first three years

I divided up the first three years with regard to learning to walk, speak and think:
1. In the course of movement development, the child forms two perception-directions and -poles: on the one hand, s/he perceives from the head, from there he takes hold of himself, and on the other, from the outside, by feeling himself. That is like a double current.
2. In the course of learning to speak, he takes hold mostly of the middle of the human being.
3. In the course of learning to think, he begins to penetrate all that lives in him with intentionality. The younger the child is, the more refined is the time-structure.

The first third of the first seven years

The first third of the first seven years can be further divided – into developmental phases of nine months:

1. Taking hold of the body

This is what it is about in the first third, in the first nine months, the focus is on taking hold of the body. This process is something generally-human. World wide it proceeds in a similar way.

2. Taking hold of speech

During the next nine months, the «middle-time» follows learning to speak. It begins world-wide with ‹ä› and ‹örö›. From this develops the individual speech. In speech development the sounding is very similar at first, although, baby-crying sounds different already, depending on the mother tongue. Babies emphasize in crying either the first or the second syllable. That means, they have taken in a rhythm. It can be observed, that a baby's muscle tone rises, when he hears a foreign language, and calms down when he hears his mother tongue.

3. Will formation

In the third part, beginning around the 19th month, the child begins to do things willingly.

I have studied development charts, and I noticed that with most empiricists, we first find months and then quarters of the year. The language used in everyday life confirms: My child is one month old, he is two months old. He is half a year old, and then he is one and a half.

Before, during pregnancy, we have nine months. That is three times three months, we speak of the first, the second and the third trimester. Anyone who was pregnant knows that these three sections feel different.

Pikler-Loczy-observation-form

I would now like to give you an example of the Pikler-Loczy Observation-sheet[1] published in the booklet *Beobachten, Verstehen und Begleiten* (Observing, Understanding, and Accompanying), and combining both.

The observation sheet represents a space-time graphic: the development goes upwards, the staircase goes upwards.

The first three years of life are depicted in five horizontal divisions, in five developmental areas:

1. The first column is the movement column. It contains criteria for the development of movement, especially for «gross motor skills». Emmi Pikler insisted not to talk about «grob-motor skills» (rough-motor skills) because motor skills are never «rough». There are «large motor skills» and there are «fine motor skills».
2. This is followed by behavior during care taking and eating, when «being together».
3. A small column stands for «cleanliness» and has a more informative character.
4. The eye-hand-coordination is anchored in fine motor skills and play activity when «being-by-oneself».
5. In the bottom column, note the vocalization and reacting to speech.

These are five big groups. The curves are above each other because several things go parallel. In the movement column are again five different criteria:

1. The child turns to the side.
2. He turns onto the belly.
3. He turns on the belly and back.
4. He rolls.
5. He crawls on belly.

The speed of development can be read from right to left – a box is provided for each month: in the left-bright area, we find one quarter of the children located at this development speed. In the dark central area, half of the children are placed. In the right area, another quarter of the children are placed.

IMPORTANT: This developmental sheet is not for children with special needs, who need different kinds of considerations.

Development speed and development phases

Mrs. Pikler and I were sitting with this sheet when it was not yet published. I described the children in the right area as «late developers». Emmi Pikler said:

---

[1] Herunterzuladen unter (download under) www.pikler.de.

We could just call them «thoroughgoing human beings».

Repeatedly she said:

Why are we not worry about the children who cannot rest and enjoy? Why do we worry about the thoroughgoing people and do not let them tap their full potential, so that they can only do everything half or three quarters?

At that time there were no ADS or ADHS. If we do not give the child time to mature in the developmental steps, s/he moves on to the next higher level with inferior prerequisites. In this respect, the sheet serves 80% of my work time as qualified reassurance for parents. I never give the sheet with the normal curve, but only one in which I enter the development of the respective child. For example, I can explain to the parents that their child is in middle-field. Or that their child is thorough, that their child waits to do something until he is sure that he can succeed.

Who decides which behavior is more intelligent?

Here is portrayed the time of the movement development, the speech development, and the relationship development in different fields. There is good empirical study material on these subjects, for, the children in the infant-care-home were demonstrably healthy, so the data are reliable. Two doctoral theses deal with the «parents' sheet». The most important feedback for me from these PhD theses was, that the parents stated that they could design the environment better and happier because they had a positive expectation.

With regard to the division into three parts of the seven year cycles, something caught my eye: If you put many curves above of each other, the early developers tend to start steeply, whereas the thoroughgoing developers start slowly. Interestingly, many development curves do not meet at two-and-a-half years, but most matches occur at two and a half months: So, with just two and a half months, many children are at the same level of development, regardless of whether they are fast-starters or thorough human beings. This suggests an underlying order and structure. Within this structure the development of the child takes place in an individual way. But here too there are exceptions.

Trouser-pocket Eurythmy

I like trouser pocket Eurythmy because we can practice everywhere without anyone noticing it. For the following exercise you only need one hand. Please close your hand like a flower bud. The young child does not yet make a fist but closes the hand like a bud. Make the bud open and close. I want to invite you now to imitate the text with one hand and then with the other:

*Alles ist im Keim enthalten,
alles Wachstum, ein Entfalten,
leises Auseinanderrücken,
dass sich einzeln könne schmücken,
was zusammen war geschoben.*

Jetzt kommt die Steigerung:

*Will am Stängel stets nach oben.
Blüt' um Blüte rücket weiter.
Sieh' es an und lern' es heiter:
zu entwickeln, zu entfalten,
was im Herzen ist enthalten!*

Approximately:
*All is in a seed contained
all the growth and all unfolding,
softly done the separating,
and each discretely decorating
which anew together came.*

Now the escalation/enhancement:
*If along the stem and ever higher
blossom after blossom upwards dance.
Do observe it, and learn gladly:
to develop, to unfold
what the heart contains untold.*

Friedrich Rückert describes what we want to observe in young children: In the first three months the arms of a child who is lying on his back are at the side of his head, and the palms of the hands are relaxed and turned heaven-wards. When he wakes up, he builds up a little tonus (muscle tension). The little arms come more together. He begins to stretch and alternately open and close his hands – and then the hand meets the mouth: The child begins to suckle on it. Suckling the hand is associated with great joy. All that can be felt there! Out of great joy there happens an all-around-stretching.

An example of observing the hand-play

I would like to continue with these small, delicate movements and look at them thoroughly together with you using an example.

– Eye-hand-coordination

It was a discovery for me to be able to see Rudolf Steiner's teaching of the senses directly on the pictures of Emmi Pikler. Exact documentation allows a deepening of everyday observation. On the other hand, it is about schooling oneself, making a connection between what you have as background knowledge and what you see. This makes it easier for us to be present in the here and now when dealing with the child.

A three-week-old boy suckles on the outside of the hand. He is already somewhat awake, otherwise he would not be sucking. The eyes are closed. The fingertips move in the direction of the mouth and the eyes open. When lips, fingertips and tongue touch, it is a sensory sensation. There are many touch receptors, and he wakes up. He wakes up and comes via the touch to experience himself. At first it is a perception: I feel myself. The nice thing about feeling is that you slip into the hand as though from inside. Now the child begins to move. By moving, he perceives the moving hand; then the eye begins to follow the hand – this shows that the eye – hand coordination begins with the sense of touch.

– Sense of movement and the formation of sounds

Subsequently the sense of movement is added and mediates between «the one who is inside», and the child's experiences. When we observe children, we can feel what at this early age is already establishing itself.

Did you ever sit by the bed of a child that happily says «örö», and shortly afterwards «fkkkkk»?

He has discovered his hand:
Where does the intensity go?
It goes into the forming of sounds of «örö», where the tonus weakens. It is as if

someone wanted to give brief greetings – and «shoo» he is gone.

It shows that there is no will, no intentionality in the hand yet. The child cannot yet take his hand and look at it. He has to conquer his limbs first from fingertips to toes via activity in the world and make it his own. It is exciting to see what helps him.

– The suckling-reflex – the primal-incarnation-muscle

I believe, the suckling reflex is the «primal-incarnation-muscle». It serves suckling. It is wonderful how a child works while he is suckling. It is visible, that breastfed children speak more articulately. I do not think it is because they have been training the muscles of the mouth while sucking. Such conclusions arise from our mechanistic thinking. Breastfed children have taken hold of their primal incarnation muscle power through sucking. They had to work hard right from the beginning: The milk did not flow to them through a large hole in the bottle so that it wouldn't take so long. When you see how quickly children become warm when they are breastfeeding, and how they taste right down to the tips of their toes, you realize that the whole muscle system is working. Then the child is not only full and warm, but also tired. Then he sleeps, grows and thrives.

– Conquering the hands via the fingertips

I am remaining now with the first quarter of the year. Let us observe a child who already opens his hand. Then the little thumb wanders between the opened lips. If you have a bit of time, you can see what can happen to you and that we are not talking about sucking as with a pacifier. Sometimes the little thumb is still in the bud – then it goes nowhere – not the child either, s/he stays outside. Then the hand is opened, because it is more interesting to taste the fingertips, and sometimes a little finger then wanders into the opened mouth – and it does not close. It only closes when he feels that there is one. This is the way that children conquer their hands calmly, slowly, taking their time. From this time onwards they become their good friends.

– Transition from being-alone to dialogue

The child is placed in the pediatrician practice on the scales, in an unfamiliar place. On the scales he is not in balance; the scales move and the adult is usually concentrated on the scale. Those who know the old scales know that they are not as light as they are today.

The child has connected with his bodily organization when he knows his hand so well, that it gives him comfort in unpleasant situations. He has a good friend with him and yet another. On each side one. In every life-situation. We can see it on the picture. One has captured the other. He holds on to it and concentrates intensely. Expressed in Eurythmy, I would say: This is the primal-A and the first E. At this moment, the child is totally present that is why he looks cross-eyed to the inside.

Everything that exists in twos now connects and begins to speak with one another. The opening and closing, the stretching still had something plant-like from the time of the being- at- one, of wholeness, for the child was one with the universe when he rested within himself.

Here the transition is taking place to the two, to the dialogue. Now we have the transition from the first quarter of the year to the second.

– World-interest – the beginning of social development –

I will show a brief film sequence of a child at the end of the first quarter of the year, after he has «wrestled» himself into his bodily organization. Children that want to feel at home in a new situation do at first what they already know from an earlier developmental phase. Only after that can they take up the new, they then do something that is new and exciting for them. When you take a child, for example, into another room, he will do things where he feels safe – because the environment has changed.

At this point therapeutic early diagnostics can begin: Some human beings incarnate in a way that they feel well enough by themselves and only come to meet the world by what passes through their fingers.

The healthy child is now at the point where he no longer has to hold onto the second hand to be sure that it does not disappear. He can manage his two hands well enough so that they stay there when he looks at them.

The next step represents for me a milestone in development. If we had our own U-books, this would be the milestone that starts social development – with world interest. The child turns the hand to the world. That is an incredible moment. I have the impression that the child gains profile at this moment. Everything that is available is taken hold of: He pulls the ribbon out of the jacket, tries to remove the veil, turns his blanket over, fiddles with the buttons and with the button hole. He takes everything and looks at it. The child turns the hand to the world.

Opening and closing was like building the inner space, a preparation for an open-minded turning to the world. Letting go and taking hold of can therefore be understood as an intensification of opening and closing.

– Movement- and rest pole

We see a boy touching a cloth. His movements still are restrained. It is exciting that both the movement pole and the rest pole develop at the same time. Every cultural movement demands also the ability to hold still.

- If, for example, you want to thread a needle and you move both the needle and the hand, it will not work.
- When cutting with knife and fork, you always have a pole of rest and a movement pole.

Movement is cultivated by the ability to restrain movement in order to be able to move purposefully. I internalize and connect what I have done in space. The many children, who are said not to have broken their reflexes at school age, stand out mainly by disturbing movements. Movement pole and resting pole belong together!

In the next picture we see the same child in the same situation, a larger movement with the cloth. Now the resting pole is not a resting pole anymore, but a balancing pole, that keeps the balance for the big movements, so that the child does not fall over.

– Hiding and finding again

The same child six weeks later: He holds the cloth confidently in both hands. The first grasping happens with the entire palm. We see one after another the grasping with the whole hand, with the middle of the hand, and then the pointed grasping with the fingertip.

In the second quarter of the year the children begin to bring something into relation. I have noticed that object permanence is not comprehended by playing with objects, but by playing with the hand: the child hides his hand, he feels it in the hiding place. Then he looks to see whether it is still there. Only much later does he hide objects. The interesting thing about the game is the hiding and the finding each other again. Children in an infant home play hide-and-seek with their caregivers at 14 or 15 months, and only from 1 3/4 years on with other children. This shows the strong connection to the adult – this is natural, to imitate the one who is adult.

With the other children they can easily play later.

– Catching up with development

Here you see what I mean when I speak of «prepared environment» for children who were not able to develop sufficiently. There are children who get a pacifier – then their little hands are left alone, they do not come to the child because they are not welcomed.

Now the question can be raised, what can we do in such a case? A ball is something the child can «grasp», can touch. Even when he is not yet adept but opens the hand and moves it, the ball remains there. He feels his fingers and there is a chance that the fingertips will meet. That would be a proposal for a child who has been prevented from experiencing everything I showed today. We must ask ourselves seriously:

How can someone act, when the precondition, the delicate finger-tip- feeling is missing?

We speak of «prepared environment» in connection with creating possibilities for the child to recover the missing development. I think it would be good for many children today, to find an environment where they can work on themselves undisturbed. Some children who grow up at home are on the go a lot and are not «at home». They are busy resettling themselves all the time, and therefore cannot work. Then they do not really get tired, but exhausted and fidgety. In this respect, the question arises, where a child can develop well and to what extent. I believe it is important to have the courage to look at every situation individually to see how and where the child can experience childhood.

A mother who cannot take being at home and goes to work, does not have to give her child away for many hours immediately. Whatever the situation is – it is most important that mother and child feel well. They are still so closely connected with one another that the child lives in the mother's atmosphere. So much for the second quarter of the year. I call it the age of the «dialogues», because the children begin to relate one object to another, and to play with the duality of the hands.

It is exciting when you look at the sleeping position. The child begins to change something here and there, and we have a premonition of the Standbein and the Spielbein: One foot goes from the middle upwards, the other one is down. After that, the children sleep on their stomach and turn the limbs earthward. That is the time, when they take hold of hands and feet and of space. Only then follows the duality in the dialogue.

Conquer greatest possible freedom

Imagine a child in stomach position. It is amazing that children conquer for themselves the greatest possible freedom on every movement-level, before they leave it. When we push them to continue, we prevent them from gaining the greatest possible freedom. This works like a damming up as far as the intentions of the child, because he is rushed to do the next thing before he could fully savor his new -found flexibility. After the hands, the feet begin to grasp, and with the grasping of the feet, in the lightness, the foot is being formed. Now the child begins to be interested in the world in all directions. He discovers the effect of himself beyond his physical limits.

It is exciting when children discover what the shadow does. I observed that with my daughter. The linen sheet was taken off and she had seen the shadow of her hand, and wanted to take it. The tonus relaxes and the hand goes between the mattress and the bed-wall. She looked for it. A child does these things until she realizes that there is a cause and an effect. After that she does not try that ever again. S/he never tries again to move the shadow, without using his hand.

Forming saturated concepts

Children continue to do something until they understand it. Then they have formed «saturated concepts», concepts, sensually saturated concepts, that are full of life and grow along with him. I noticed that there are steps. We can recognize something, we can grasp it, and we can understand it. We have a separate word for each of these areas:
- recognize
- grasp
- understand

After one object come two objects and finally the whole world comes into conversation. Dialogue is followed by an engagement with several objects, with the world, with sound, with noise and with forms. Children never tire of picking up different things. In the third quarter of the year, we can observe how the hand, gliding over the form of the object, adjusts itself to how it should be grasped. Children do not tire during this time to lift something and let it drop again. To explore that something flat and round dances, something else rolls away, and how a little building block stays in its place.

Own observing

Concerning the development Janusz Korczak writes: «The book with the finished forms has dulled the gaze and made thinking lazy. Living by the observations, experiences and opinions of others, trust in ourselves has been lost so much, that we no longer want to see from our own perspective anymore. As if the printed word were a revelation and not the product of research by some other human being, just not my own, aimed somewhere at some human being, only not today and at my own child.»[2]

How does this role model seem to you? Do you feel how the inquiring, interested adult in you is just as active as the child?

Those who only wait for milestones, for what is not happening, they do something else. As a rule, we have check-and-read-care children in Germany through surveys, for example, if we think of the language skill surveys and to the first grade readiness examinations.

*Are we asking the right questions, the right questions at the right time?
Who tests?
Who decides?*

I would like to leave these questions in the room.

Observation – Respect

I am now going back to the one who observes and the one who is his role model. The word «observation – (Beobachtung)» contains the word «respect – (Achtung)». We can hear respect in different ways. Respect can have something to do with awe: «I'll sit back and make room for you». But it can also mean: pay attention, «Watch out, you dummy!»

How I use words depends on how they came to meet me. Whether they hurt me or not. So the question is:

*How am I looking?
What is my task?*

It is not up to parents to diagnose. Diagnosis is the task of the doctors. We expect more from professional educators and rightly so, than from parents, a little more experience and insight into how development takes place. Steiner left an unbelievable amount on this topic. I have searched for a long time, how we can reach this respect, this mindfulness that we hear about everywhere and that we demand. Mindfulness comes as a quality from Buddhism. If you say to a head-man, «be mindful!» then he'll pay attention, and try to watch well.

Piaget[3] described how he had a writing pad and pencil ready and looked expectantly at the child. The child folded his arms

---

[2] Janusz Korczak, * 22. Juli 1878 in Warsaw; † after 5. August 1942 presumably in the Treblinka extermination camp, was a Polish physician, and author of children's books and important pedagogue.

[3] Jean Piaget was Professor of Psychology at the university of Geneva from 1929 to 1954 and founder of the Centre International d'Épistémologie, also in Geneva. He also held a Professorship at the University of Neuchâtel and at the Sorbonne in Paris.

and looked back at him expectantly. The imitation ability was intact. Then both were waiting. Piaget quickly realized that it is better when a child is in his familiar environment, when the mother, for example, is ironing in the background. He then observed casually through a hatch of the kitchen. This is how he researched.

I have tried for myself to seek how we can come to mindfulness, if it is a heart virtue. I would like to read to you now the Ecce Homo (5) from the *Truth-Wrought-Words* by Steiner. I would like to convey to you, how you can weave different ways of respecting into what we think, what we feel and what we will, in order not to get hung up on images or to expect something to happen in the child's development. It will happen the moment you need to go to the toilette and you are not watching. Then the child is free.

Ecce Homo
In the heart the weaving feeling,
This concerns the dialogue time, the duality, the middle
In the head the light of thinking,
In the limbs the strength of willing.
Here we are in mindfulness:
Feeling can connect with thinking and willing
Weaving enlightening,
Strengthening weaving,
Enlightened strengthening:
Lo! This is man.[4]

We need to do something with ourselves to be mindful and aware. So that we do not just «watch» or «lie in wait». We cannot look into the heavens in these times, but only look into others. However, if you look in the above mentioned way, you will receive incredibly gifts.

---

4 Rudolf Steiner, *Truth Wrought Words*. GA 40. Translation: Arvia MacKaye Ege.

Helmuth von Kügelgen (†)
To receive the child with reverence![1]

*The healthy social life is found
when in the mirror of each human soul
the whole community finds its reflection,
and when in the community
the virtue of each one is living.*
Rudolf Steiner[2]

Why paint an ideal when reality gives us a different picture?

Two- and three-year-olds are torn out of the enfoldment of the protective care – here out of need, there out of necessity from the perspective of social and societal conditions, or because adults give priority to their own needs and destinies. But even from the mother's physical protective sheath they are already ripped out and may not continue the connection of being and embodiment in life.

Who has the right to judge the intimate, individual decisions that other people have made for themselves?

It cannot be the task of the kindergarten teacher, the Waldorf educator, to take the conviction, that he has struggled to achieve as consciously and independently as possible, to the parental homes in a missionary way. We do not have to bless or moralize the single parent, we have to help him/her! From the beginning! Even through the education of the youngest, through social arrangements, through changes in political and economic and social conditions. Perhaps one day, we will look at the world from the needs of the children, then there will be a very different behavior by the adults, when they understand that after birth, children still need sheaths from us three more times, until they have found themselves completely.

But the actual incarnation sheath is needed by the children of the first seven years, when they are passing from the hand of the angel into the hand of the «caregiver».

Do we not have to help children who are otherwise only looked after?
Are we only talking to mothers and fathers when we take care of their children?
Can social welfare stations, children's crèches and so on not just as likely become cultural centers from which emanate ideas and concrete social changes?

However they may be designed, they should help children to incarnate in a healthy way and lead more and more adults to respect human dignity, which should not only be focused on heroes, superiors and loved ones, but on every child as well. «*Accept the child with reverence*» is a formulation by Rudolf Steiner for the body forming education in the first seven years. No theoretically calculated opening hours of the kindergarten, no daily activity schedules, no holiday schedules and no breakfast plan are the necessary consequence of this protection forming reverence. Which doll, which colors, which toys – everything depends on the attitude of the educator that forms relationships. This is a creative process: From the forces and possibilities of the educator, from the perception of the concrete children, who come from their and not from an imaginary environment,

---

[1] Exerpt from an essay, Spring 1991 in the 9. Rundbrief der Internationalen Vereinigung der Waldorfkindergärten.
[2] Rudolf Steiner, *Truth Wrought Words*, GA 40.

«education as an art» has to develop. Certainly it is not arbitrary! Your constant teacher and counselor, your source of inspiration and creative educator's imagination is – in addition to love for the child and his perception – the study of the human being's soul-spiritual- and bodily- nature. All models and methods which the beginner first follows and which protect the experienced educator from falling into routine must be thought over and examined from time to time. If I struggle again and again with older boys, I have to change my pedagogical approach, and not get rid of the boys or «suffer» forever. If I cannot live up to children's needs, if they go hungry in any field of life, of play, of work in the kindergarten, then I lack imagination.

Waldorf education, the art of education, is not a program; it must find different answers to social, societal, and human conditions. For every emerging question, a joint searching, a real conversation between kindergarten teacher, parents and board of trustees has to begin. On the subject of «longer opening hours» e.g. any partner could quickly propose a simple solution to the problem: the kindergarten teacher should stay longer, says the board. Another teacher should be hired, say the parents. The parents should work less and care more about their children ... No! Such increase of extra work here or there, does not help, neither does moral preaching nor blaming others. Out of the need of the situation, the carrying strength must be developed, which leads to more money, more joy in working, to changes in social conditions, and so on. Money for personnel and space expansion is not easily obtained. Even non-profit is becoming ever tighter and the laws are making it difficult for us. The general social conditions, the occupational situations, the demands for a living standard, the brutal economic need, the views of what is necessary for a living – all this is not easy to change; and we do not only want children of an elite group, a mix of money and conviction. The kindergarten teacher extends her work for several hours and foregoes part of her salary so that an additional room can be rented or remodeled.

The pedagogical profession has the peculiarity that at the same point, namely in human relationships, enormous powers are either given or wasted. What a source of strength, life, and imagination, is a warm-hearted, friendly relationship between educators, children, parents, and the board! If it has cooled, and the joy in each other is gone, the trust disturbed, then the forces run off like water from the hole in the bucket. Just as there are difficult children, there are also difficult board members or difficult parents and, of course, difficult educators. Yet! The one has to carry the burden of the other; then forces arise, then imagination develops into new possibilities. It can be found in any field – no matter if it is about money, strength of commitment, or an attitude of service – solutions can be found or at least initiated when working together. But only when the tasks of the whole kindergarten community – the parents, the children, the educators, the board – are mirrored in the soul of the individual, will each individual be warmed in his initiative, and his power will become fruitful in the community: «*The healthy social life is found when in the mirror of each human soul the whole community finds its reflection ...*» We should not shy away from questioning all habits, and we should ask ourselves:

What is necessary today?

What is tried and tested needs the power of a new decision, the necessary new ideas need prudence before we seek to realize them and make a decisions. We do not only need love for children but also love for the educators' work, with all its challenges.

We do not only need to be happy that we have a kindergarten, but also love to work on social questions, and on the emerging future forms and ideas. We do not only need money, but also the love for ways in which new little rivulets are created into which money will want to flow. An inexhaustible source of power flows when we work together, in cooperation, willing to accept the initiative of the individual, and keeping in mind that the conversation of two, three or more people must prepare the space, so that He can be in the midst of us, whom we already take in as child at Christmas in reverence and love.

Claudia Grah-Wittich and Brigitte Huisinga
The pedagogical impulse of Emmi Pikler and Waldorf education

Emmi Pikler was born in Vienna in 1902 and died in 1984 in Budapest. She studied medicine in Vienna and received her pediatric specialist-training with Freiherr Clemens von Pirquet. As a teacher, he shaped her later life's task, for, he took the approach that medically it is first of all necessary, to keep the child healthy and «not to limit oneself to the detection and cure of illnesses. Not the illness was the main thing, but the child.»[1] Pirquet occupied himself intensively with educational questions. Training in the «Pirquet-Clinic» naturally included internship for the care and nutrition of the baby.

Thanks to another teacher, the pediatric surgeon Hans Salzer, Emmi Pikler learned how very different an examination proceeds when the doctor turns to the little patients in a friendly manner, and builds up a good contact with them. Both impulses, the education for health and prevention in the sense of Pirquet as well as the empathetic attitude of Salzer towards the child, influenced Emmi Pikler's later own approach. Important on her professional path was also her own husband, who as a mathematician and pedagogue shared her considerations in developmental-physiology. Both of them decided at the birth of their first child to do everything possible to enable their child to develop in a healthy way – to respect the child's own developmental dynamics and to accompany him/her with patience and not to restrict the free movement development.

From 1935 onwards Emmi Pikler was recognized and active in Hungary as a pediatrician. She gave lectures on the care and raising of infants and young children and worked for ten years as family doctor in her private practice. After the war, she took care of abandoned and malnourished children within a Hungarian organization. In 1946 she founded the home for infants Lóczy.

Thanks to the carefully guided care-givers and the mindful design of the environment, she managed to create an atmosphere of security in which the children could grow up without developing the usual signs of neglect or hospitalism.

Emmi Pikler tirelessly researched and observed the children in her practice. From these child observations, she developed her own differentiated approach to the child's independent movement-development.

The pedagogical impulse of Emmi Piklers focuses mainly to three aspects:

1. Care of the child
This is about the «being together» of adults and children. The adults must insure that it happens in good harmony. Inner peace, and a high level of presence in all care-takers' activities are part of the natural understanding of Pikler's pedagogy. All actions are done in amicable contact with the child.

2. Free movement development
The basic need of every child to do everything themselves and to try it out, is deliberately given space. In this way a free

---

[1] Emmi Pikler, *Laßt mir Zeit! (Don't rush me)* 3. ed. 2001.

development of movement is made possible and concomitantly the free unfolding of each child according to his individual time rhythms.

3. Forming the environment
Deliberately forming the environment creates an atmosphere of security for the free play and the care of the children.

Emmi Pikler's pedagogical insights are based on a wealth of perceptions that show a variety of developmental possibilities – which is why Pikler resolutely distances herself from all infant development programs and standards.

As part of her research, she found out through close observation that children who are given the necessary free space by adults, develop according to their inherent laws. The prerequisites are that the adult is present and has a good relationship with the children. The language that he uses to accompany all actions has a supportive effect: these are not explanations, questions or teachings, but rather descriptions of what the hands do.

Emmi Pikler's research results and Waldorf education
If we place the findings and observations of Emmi Pikler in relation to anthroposophic understanding of the human being, the following can be stated:
- Emmi Pikler's studies on children's autonomous movement development are based on exact observation of children, and complement the understanding of the human being inspired by spiritual science.
- Both approaches do not measure the development of the child in terms of external standards and programs. Rather, they are based on the inherent law of development of the child.
- Both approaches attach the greatest importance to the form and design of the environment as an important point of reference for child development. Rudolf Steiner emphasizes what Emmi Pikler suggests: «*Only the right physical environment affects the child so that his physical organs are shaped in the right way.*»[2]
- In both approaches, adults are decisive as role models, which the child needs for his development for orientation and imitation.
- Both approaches consider free play, where educators should not interfere, decisive for the development.
  – Pikler fights for free movement development as essential for the overall development of the child.
  – Rudolf Steiner emphasizes the importance of free movement development as prerequisite and preparation for the development of speaking and thinking and the development of self-consciousness.

From her examinations and findings, Emmi Pikler built up a school for toddler- or elementary education, and the contents are today received with great interest by educated pedagogical circles.

---

[2] Rudolf Steiner, *The Education of the Child in the light of Anthroposophy*. GA 34. Dornach 1969.

Brigitte Huisinga

Where do we take children below three?

In a city like Frankfurt it is quite natural today that a young child does not grow up at home anymore, but in some facility or with a day-mother, who cares for him/her at times.

Several arguments are used to justify this development:
- early education
- concern for the future professional career of the child
- the widespread opinion that a little one has to acquire already very early social competence in a children's group.

On the other hand, there are life situations of various kinds that require childcare: these can be economic or social reasons, also overburdening or isolation of mother or father or educational insecurity and other worries.

I would like to pursue the following questions:

Do children need an infant care facility for the first three years?

Is there anything missing for their development, if they grow up in their own home during this time?

– Reasons for growing up in the family

From the point of view of Waldorf education, it is easy to answer that growing up in one's own family, when the family can afford it and none of the afore-mentioned conditions speak against it, offers the healthiest prerequisites for the child's development: the child learns to walk, speak and think in the security and in close connection with his parents who lovingly care for him. The child can observe them in the daily household activities and imitate them, he has their support and backing in all his experiences. The family is a group also and is therefore a small social network, in which the child can learn living in togetherness with other people.

A decisive step in the development takes place around the third year of life. Now he has become more independent in many actions. He can eat independently, he can make himself understood, he does not need, or soon will not need any diapers anymore. He clearly says «I», indicating that he can distinguish his own person from other people. Now he wants to try himself out, even in a group with other children, and he slowly is getting mature enough for this.

– Reasons for a day nursery

Going to a day nursery is not the child's need. To put a child into a day nursery is a need of the parents or a necessity that needs to be respected and supported in the present time, whether the reasons are isolation, a career, financial, or personal. If the mother feels that she cannot stay home, providing childcare is often helpful to both child and mother. Crucial is the quality of the relationship between mother and child when they are together. If they enjoy being together, then a day nursery whose employees are aware of the great responsibility of this task can even support home care and up-bringing.

What conditions does a day nursery have to fulfill so that children do not only survive without harm but even benefit from it?

Before we opened the first group of the «Wiegestube Sonnenschein» in 2002, we were concerned with the question what form of care on the basis of Waldorf education would corresponds to the developmental needs of children, and not just a kindergarten in miniature form. Here we were helped by the experience and research of the Pikler Institute in Budapest, with which we had been familiar for many years through advanced training and internships. The correspondences and additions to Waldorf education gave us the courage to venture on this task of an infant care facility which is increasingly demanded by society.

Requirements for a healthy development in an infant care facility:
1. regulated daily routine
2. mindful care and free activity
3. professional attitude
4. time for familiarization and bonding.

1. Regulated daily routine
The daily routine must be clearly structured according to the needs of the children – this gives them orientation and security. No child should live in uncertainty when, for example, the outdoor play time takes place, when he will get something to eat, etc., and that he can also be sure to be picked up again by his family.

A well-regulated daily routine not only gives orientation to the children but also makes the work easier for the caregivers. The simple processes become a matter of course for both sides, whereby every rhythm and every order must permit variations if necessary.

2. Mindful care and free activity
It may seem strange to address these two issues together. According to the research of the Pikler Institute in Budapest, the attentive, warm contact of the caregiver during the care is a precondition for the child's autonomous activity, and for his interest in the environment.

The care area is separated from the play area by a lattice, so that the care can proceed undisturbed, without the care-giver losing sight of the other children. At the same time, the playing children see the adults as active humans. The activity encourages them via imitation to their own activity.

The children are diapered in rotating order one after the other and, if necessary, also in between, of course. Each child has a primary caregiver, who helped him settle in and who puts his diapers on at least once a day, and closely monitors and tracks his development.

Mindful care
What does mindful care mean to us?
From the beginning, the child is treated as an individual, competent personality, who gives us signals about her well-being. With calm, loving language, the actions to be carried out with child are prepared, and she is given time to participate. In this way, she will gradually participate more and more actively. The caregiver gives her whole attention to the child and perceives how she feels, and what she needs. Putting diapers on, is a joyous togetherness. Usually, diapers are changed with children lying on their backs. From a certain time of

development onwards this no longer corresponds to their need for movement. The children turn or stand up later. In order not to force her on her back against her impulse, the diaper changing station must be designed accordingly with safety in mind. A lattice protects the children, gives them freedom of movement and relieves the caregiver of the worry that they might fall off. Even in these changed positions, the dialogue with the child is not interrupted. It is always a great pleasure to experience when a child begins to reach out to us with her arm, or when standing, stretch a leg toward us.

This mindful care requires a high level of perceptiveness and presence of the educator, which requires professional practice. Not to let your thoughts digress, to be fully present, let quiet gentle hands speak to the child through gestures, lovingly accompany all doing, telling the child what will be done now, but also responding to the gestural and vocal sounds of the child. This kind of affection causes the child to show satisfaction after the care, so that she can now explore her environment with interest. To put it in Emmi Pikler's words: The child is «satiated of being together» and now wants to be «alone».

Under the aspect of sensory development and sensory care, this «being together» with the caregiver is of great importance, especially for the sense of life and the sense of touch. The quality with which we touch the child is crucial and has a great deal to do with feeling at home in the body. Henning Köhler speaks about the «gentle certainty», when we treat the child.

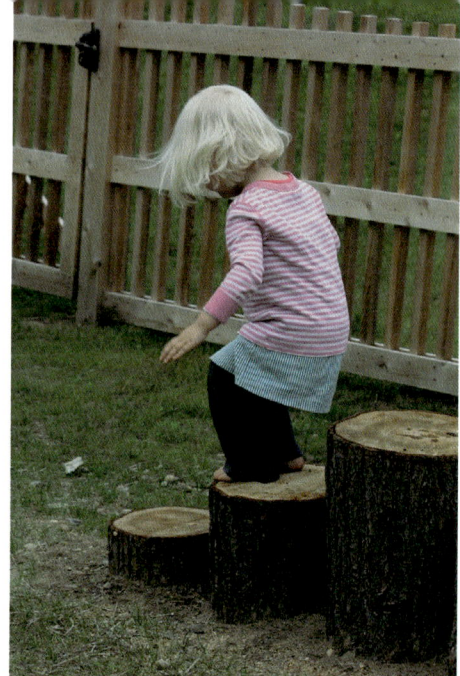

Fig. 1

This includes respecting the differences of children according to their age, constitution, and sensitivities.

Free activity in play and movement

The times between the care situations, the changing of diapers, dressing and undressing, eating and sleeping are available to the children for free play. However, they also want to be perceived in their engagement: The caregiver keeps looking over to them again and again and keeps an eye on conflict situations. In particular, she enjoys the children's activities.

The observations and insights of Emmi Pikler guide us in the care, when they learn to eat by themselves as well as with the autonomous development of movement. We do not bring the children into positions they cannot yet acquire by themselves (such as lying on their stomach or propping them up in a sitting position), and do not carry them when they can reach a destination themselves (like climb-

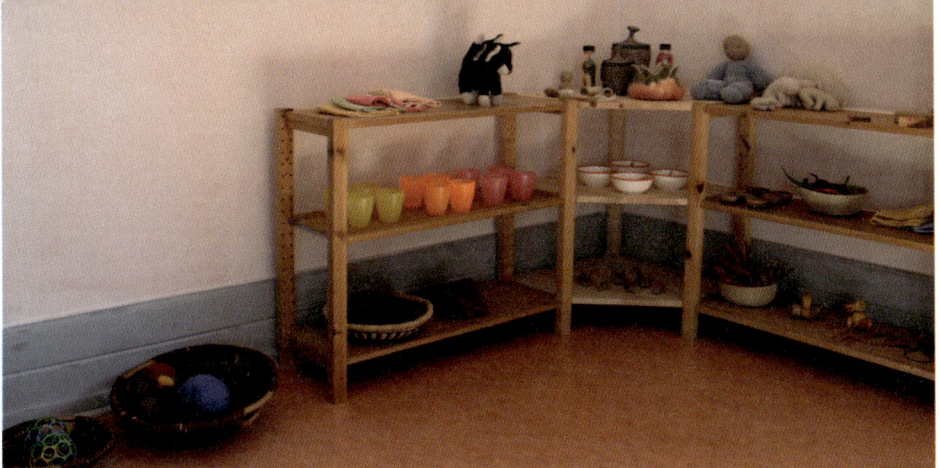

Fig. 2

ing stairs) we make sure that no dangerous situations arise.

Children are looking for movement challenges, for example, on stairs or tree trunks and try them out by themselves. Again and again, we can observe that they only expect of themselves what they feel they can do. They are happy when they have succeeded. Often they look to make sure, we have seen it too.

There too, a respectful, joyful look is enough and they feel perceived and confirmed.

Depending on the development, the other play materials such as building blocks, cloths, mugs, pots, simple dolls or buckets serve for the touching and exploring of the physical laws and the order of the world, in symbolic play and, with increasing age, for an imaginative reproduction of everyday life and experiences. In play and movement, the child learns to know himself and the laws of the world. In the self-chosen experiments, the child not only learns how the objects behave, but learns to endure when something does not succeed immediately. Perseverance and tireless practice lead to success – an experience that the child takes along for his entire life.

Free play and the development of movement would merit a separate article from the point of view of the development and care of the senses. All four body-senses are addressed here most strongly.

3. Professional attitude

The always repeated succession of activities appears to be trivial and simple, but on the other hand it places a high demand on the person in charge.

The recurring simplicity harbors the danger of routine, the requirement for perception the danger of being overwhelmed. And one more thing: The little child addresses the maternal feelings of the educator and transference can occur. She learns to love «her» designated child, likes to hold her in her arms, possibly jealously watches over the child. This is where self-education begins: the caregivers must learn to observe, illuminate and consciously deal with these feelings. This can only be achieved by developing a trusting, non-competitive, open relationship with the faculty where it is possible to exchange ideas, talk about everything, and help one another. Maria Vincze from the Pikler-Institute differentiates between motherly love and professional love.

Every mother raises her child in her own way, according to her feelings, and to her best knowledge and conviction. This is her prerogative. It is her child. The caregiver must not give in to her feelings. The child entrusted to her is not her own. She has to learn this difficult profession, that makes demands on body, soul and spirit. Only if she succeeds, will the children in her care develop unhindered, feel well. ... This profession requires a long, varied learning process.[1]

According to the remarks by Maria Vincze's, I will mention in the following, a few aspects that make this professional approach to the children possible.

The prerequisite is the enjoyment of the work that happens when the educator can turn with real interest to the child and perceives him in his individuality. «*Every child is extremely interesting*».[2] Over time, it will become better and better, not to wait for the progress in the child's development. It is rather about observing the smallest steps, but also about observing why a child may take a step backward, to understand this, and to accompany the child with trust when he is overcoming difficulties. However, a sound knowledge of the development of young children is the basis for seeing the individual aspect of every single child.

To summarize, professionalism, that is, knowledge combined with the willingness to engage in reflection and self-education, makes the care of young children a very interesting, fulfilling task, and prevents the caregivers from transferences.

4. Time for familiarization and bonding

The time for familiarization is a very sensitive phase for child, mother and educator, a time of uncertainty, of strong feelings, and of getting to know one another. Some days mother or father are present for hours. Over the next two or three weeks, they will gradually extend the length of time that they leave the child in the care facility. The care activities are gradually taken over by the designated caregiver for the child. But the mother has a lot of opportunity to observe the processes, the play of the children and the care giving practices. The educator attends to the mother and is in conversation with her. Trust grows and makes it easier for the mother to give her little child into someone else's hands.

A successful settling-in period, which may even take longer than three weeks, is the best prerequisite for a trusting harmony between the two sides now responsible for the well-being of the child.

– Maternal love

From the beginning of the familiarization, a distinction is made between the relationship with the mother and the relationships that arise in the institution. The care should support the child's ability to bond and not lead to psychological problems by the daily changing caregivers.

According to Myriam David, there «grows between each mother and her baby, a network of a specific, individual interaction patterns, that is very rich in every

---

1 Maria Vincze, *Mütterliche Liebe – Professionelle Liebe*. München 2002, p. 8. (Maternal Love, Professional Love)
2 Ibid.

> mother-child duality, that no other adult can achieve. ... Even if this care should be imperfect, there is a rich interaction through facial expressions and gestures, in which each partner affects the other and adapts to the other. The feeling of belonging together arises. The maternal relationship is, of course, unique and irreplaceable.»[3]

The relationship with the caregiver cannot replace this maternal relationship. If she is not aware of this and ties the child in «motherly love» to herself, she will raise false expectations in the child that cannot be fulfilled in the group. Unequal treatment of the children, guilty conscience, separation pain and competition with the parents cause problems for the educator, the parents, the group and the colleagues.

– Professional love

As already described above, the unreflected feelings can be replaced by a love that is supported by the interest of the child's wellbeing. Even the smallest child is a human partner who must be met with dignity and empathy.

> The artist, the good craftsman, looks with satisfaction and joy – we can also say with love – at the work of art he created with his hands, the successful creation. The caregiver also experiences such joy when, thanks to her care, she can discover something new every day in the development of the child. But unlike the successful piece of work, the child does not only «pay» with his thriving, but also with his love, and his affection.[4]

For us this means that in a successful caring situation, the child can additionally engage in relationships beyond that with his parents and experience no irritation that leads to insecure attachment behavior with later problems. Well-accustomed children devote themselves after the morning's separation pain to play and to the other children and turn in difficult situations to the adults. They know who their main caregiver is and are eager to get comforted by her, but they are well able to accept the other care persons. They are looking forward to the reunion with the parents. This is particularly evident when the children talk about who will pick them up, when changing diapers after their nap, whether father or mother or possibly one of their grandparents. They listen to those arriving, recognize the voices, and a radiance comes over their face. The babies stretch out their arms towards their mother, want to get to her, looking for the bodily closeness, that only comes about in this way between the parents and their children. Despite the free, active, relaxed behavior of the children during the care phase, the attachment to the parents is not impaired.

---

[3] Ibid, p.12.

[4] Ibid, p.17.

Ina von Mackensen
Familiarization in the Nursery (Crèche)

In Waldorf education familiarization and relationship building have been integrated for years, and are an integral part of the concept. Now it is also increasingly implemented in public facilities.

If you take the soul-spiritual development of the young child seriously, you have to take into account the very close connection in this age group between the child and his parents. Out of his own initiative, the young child would not want to spend several hours away from his parents on a regular basis.

As care takers, we must accept that parents find it necessary or feel that they need to have their child cared for before s/he is three. Only in this way can we accompany the children well and help them to master the great challenge.

The basis of every art of education is the unobstructed view of the needs of the incarnating child. Nevertheless, we must also include the biographical reality of today's parents who carry the responsibility for the birth and raising of the child.

Every adaptation process is a miracle: we offer a relationship, and it is open how it will develop, if we give the child the free space to contribute creatively and decisively.

I. Principles of Developmental Psychology – The Bonding Theory

The center of developmental psychology today is again the attachment theory. It is about the fundamental approach that a human being must have a secure attachment to an adult at the beginning of his childhood as a stable emotional starting point, that enables him to turn to the world creatively, with curiosity and interest. Safe bonding does not guarantee soul health and also does not protect against traumas, strokes of fate or difficult life situations. However, it creates a positive basic constitution that has been proven to increase resilience (inner strength and resistance in overcoming difficult life situations). The brain researcher Gerald Hüther formulates it as follows:

Every child needs the feeling of warm caring and security to be able to assess new situations not as a threat but as a challenge. Both exist only in the intensive relationship with other people, and it is the early psychosocial experiences made in these relationships and rooted in the child's brain that determine his further development and guide his feelings, thoughts, and actions.[1]

Secure attachment has four requirements:
1. continuous presence of an empathic caregiver
2. sensitive handling
3. appropriate reactions
4. prompt response to the needs expressed by the child.

All four categories must be continually adapted to the child's level of development.

In attachment theory three types of binding are distinguished:
1. securely attached
2. insecure, avoiding attachment
3. insecure, ambivalent attachment

---

[1] Karl Gebauer / Gerald Hüther, *Kinder brauchen Wurzeln. Neue Perspektiven für eine gelingende Entwicklung.* (Children need to have Roots. New Perspectives for a successful Development)

Even though «secure attachment» is a kind of developmental goal, the other two types of attachment (uncertain, avoiding and uncertain, ambivalent attachment) do not represent a clinical picture of illness.

– Securely attached children

can express their separation pain by crying. They are able to build a close relationship with a new caregiver on a secure basis during their parents' absence. They clearly have tantrums, show a great willingness to cooperate, and like to engage in dialogue or play. Their language is colorful and their ideas for play are imaginative.

– Children are insecure, avoiding attachment

They seem less needy and are often rewarded in our present day culture. They create less stress in the familiarization phase, but are actually under constant stress. They make a pleasant, adapted impression on the educator, are easy to guide, because they are interested in the activity of the adults. In fact, their adaptability is the inability to articulate that they miss the main caregiver. They have learned that grief, fear, anger have no place in forming a relationship with the caregiver, but adaptability and «emotional needlessness» is showered with praise.

Even though these children manage the acclimatization phase very quickly and without any problems, their stress can be physiologically verified in increased heart rate and increased Cortisol-level (detectable hormone that is released by stress).

– Children's ambivalent attachment

In the forming of the relationship, they have gone through strongly changing closeness-distance experiences, where the needs of the child were not in the foreground, but the emotional mood of the mother. They can not immerse themselves in play, because they connect their play activity constantly to the emotional reaction of the care-taker. In the good bye situations in kindergarten, these children can be recognized by the fact that they cannot detach themselves from their parents and can also not be comforted.

The forms of attachment mentioned, describe a lifelong developmental psychological imprinting of the children. However, as early attachment experiences can also be corrected, one of the main tasks of educational work is the conscious handling of the different types of children. Also grandparents, teachers and in later life, also partnerships, as well as the psychotherapy can broaden the attachment pattern.

II. The knowledge of the human being in Waldorf education

Apart from the basic developmental psychological situation in which a child grows up, Waldorf education raises the question which karmic constellation moved the individuality of the young child to place himself into this particular life situation. As educators, we try to find out carefully which being has decided to come to us.

We try as educators to create a space so the child can unfold his personality, and can take hold of his development in the first seven-year-cycle in accordance with his individuality. For we do not see the human being primarily as a «product» of environmental influences, but understand him as an individuality who has set out to take hold of and develop his instrument, the inherited body. Although we endeavor to be worthy role models, we have no influence on the individual characteristics of a child.

III. Familiarization

A. The child

Every separation situation causes separation pain, that wakes us up. With regard to the «dreaming consciousness» of the little child, it is necessary to arrange the familiarization so that the child succeeds in establishing a bond with the educating persons, and in gaining confidence and trust in order to be separated from the parents without being pushed too much into the awakening-process. Reliably recurring, predictable, ritualistic events dampen the inevitable «wake-up pain» to a degree appropriate to the child's consciousness. This process determines the dyadic relationship between the child and the care person, whereby the empathic, appreciative relationship with the parents is a support. The child's mind can confidently lean on this.

We form the acclimation gentle so that the child can find the path via trust, and not via intellectual explanations. We take time until the child is confident that his parents will always come back. This trust must be nonverbally strengthened by us as security and hope. We name and accompany the process with words that convey confidence to the child, but we ask little, do not teach, and do not explain in an abstract way. His sense of self grows out of trust and the complete connection with his environment.

A strong support comes from individual rituals that one finds as a new caregiver with the child, and senses from him/her what fits well. Whether it's a little ball game, looking for a particular cup for playing in the sand, a form of shoe cleaning accompanied by sounds, a joint look through the window of a kindergarten group – which fits very well if in that group happens to be an older sibling.

In the course of the relationship building there is often a crisis, an irritation, a dry spell. The child who, after the gentle beginning, was beaming and turning towards the new caregiver now realizes, when the separation from the primary caregiver takes place regularly, that the new relationship is not entirely determined by his own interest, but that he needs to cooperate. In this worsening crisis, the caregiver has to maintain continuously a non-coercive, unclouded offer of the relationship, in order to win the young child for this «freedom in separation». If this process succeeds, the relationship often deepens. This new relational quality is strongly influenced by the child: clear eye contact, searching for the new caregiver, but also the first touching contact and other small signs of coming closer, show, that he is ready to walk this path with us.

The familiarization process can be described as successfully completed by the child when, in difficult situations such as falling down or hurting himself, s/he calls for the caregiver and lets himself be comforted by her. But also, when he successfully copes with challenges, when something succeeds or is fun, and the child spontaneously turns to the new caregiver. Only now has the bonding process reached the necessary maturity.

There is no ideal point in time for this familiarization process. Nevertheless, when closely observing the state of development of the toddler and incorporating the findings from developmental psychology, we should pay attention to the difference in the burdening for the child, which this familiarization can bring at the respective stages of development.

Although it seems straightforward and least difficult to accustom children already in the first year of life, still the question arises, whether this is due to the fact that children at this age neither have the maturity nor the ability to express the fears and difficulties that they have. An eight-week-old infant looks forward to every smiling face.

Settling children in the defiant phase is problematic because, on the one hand, they run the risk of experiencing the event as a rejection by the parental basis, and on the other, because of their aspirations for autonomy at this age, they find it particularly difficult to make new relationships.

Each institution has to decide at what age it will take in children, in accordance with the needs of the parents and their own personal, spatial and financial possibilities.

B. The Parents

It is important to develop a separate, differentiated acclimatization concept in every child care facility, and to present it to the parents before accepting the child. Then, it is good to look together with them at their needs and at the individual situation of the child, in order to be able to customize the acclimatization process.

A prerequisite for a success of the familiarization process is the establishment of a trusting relationship between parents and educators. Even though the parents have decided to place their child into an infant care facility, it is a good bye process that is accompanied by ambivalent feelings among many parents. If the parents experience that competition is not the issue, but that with the caretaker the circle that earnestly strives to improve the well-being and development of the child has been enlarged, the foundations have been laid for successful familiarization. The home visit is a clear sign for parents and children that we as educators are concerned with an empathic relationship.

C. The educators

Getting new children accustomed is a tremendous challenge for the educators. This process is exciting, but also exhausting, because it requires a sensitive perception of the needs of everyone: I open myself, I look forward to the new parents and even more to the new child and how the relationship between us will turn out. It takes a lot of peace and serenity to be able to withstand the rejection of the child, but also to be able to endure the ambivalence of the parents in the separation process. Even though I see it as my task to shape this process, the child, the parents and the already existing group determine it as well.

It can be a relief if the group consists of several age-levels and the older children in the group already have a certain stability. Nevertheless, we as educators have to take special care of ourselves, so that we can transmit the emotional security that is necessary for this process. Self-care generally plays an important role in the profession of educators, but is especially important in this situation and requires conscious forming. A good support can be given by the group of colleagues, but also a Balint-group and/or supervision can be helpful.

Brigitte Huisinga
The Course of the day in the infant care: Wiegestube am «hof»

What should the daily rhythm look like for young children? Why is this even a question?

For a Waldorf pedagogical kindergarten, rhythm and repetition are basic elements of the daily schedule, in which there are a series of rituals like finger plays, singing games, eating together at the big table to name just a few.

What do young children need?

In the following shall be clarified why a transfer of the kindergarten does not work. For example, separation from parents for the young child in the first three years takes a much greater effort, that neither correspond to his level of development nor to his need. It is easier for a child of kindergarten age.

Unlike infants, children of kindergarten age have achieved a degree of independence – they can communicate with each other, do not need diapers anymore and organize play together with other children. The basic pedagogical situations are fundamentally different, which is why recourse to the daily design and schedule of the kindergarten is problematic for nursery institutions.

Several articles in this book describe in detail the prerequisites for infant care in order to meet the basic needs of children for food and sleep, but also for relationship and autonomy. It is not only about reducing the stress factors that are the result of separation – increase in stress hormones and sinking of growth hormones, increased susceptibility to infection – but also that the child can benefit from the care – especially in the today's time.

The design of the daily rhythm in the crèche must be considered in two main ways:
1. from the perspective of the needs of the child
2. from the perspective of the caregivers in the sense of support to cope with the challenging task of looking after young children.

1. The daily rhythm from the point of view of the child's needs

First, the needs of the child will be discussed.

Individual care for each child, where we deal and communicate respectfully with each other takes *time and space*. Likewise, the independent play of the child requires *time and space*, as well as meals, sleep and play in the fresh air.

Adults connect «time» with basic patterns of past, present and future. They are focused on a goal, must be «finished», and are under time pressure or the time does not pass, when they are waiting for something or when routine activities become boring.

Children, on the other hand, experience time differently.

Children live above all in the presence and love repetition. This is a graphic picture from an article in the Family Handbook of the state-institute for Early Childhood Education by Michael Schnabel: He sees the time for the little child as a circle, a picture that is very familiar to them – time is something repetitive. He writes:

«They are virtually rooted with this time format, because right from the first stir-

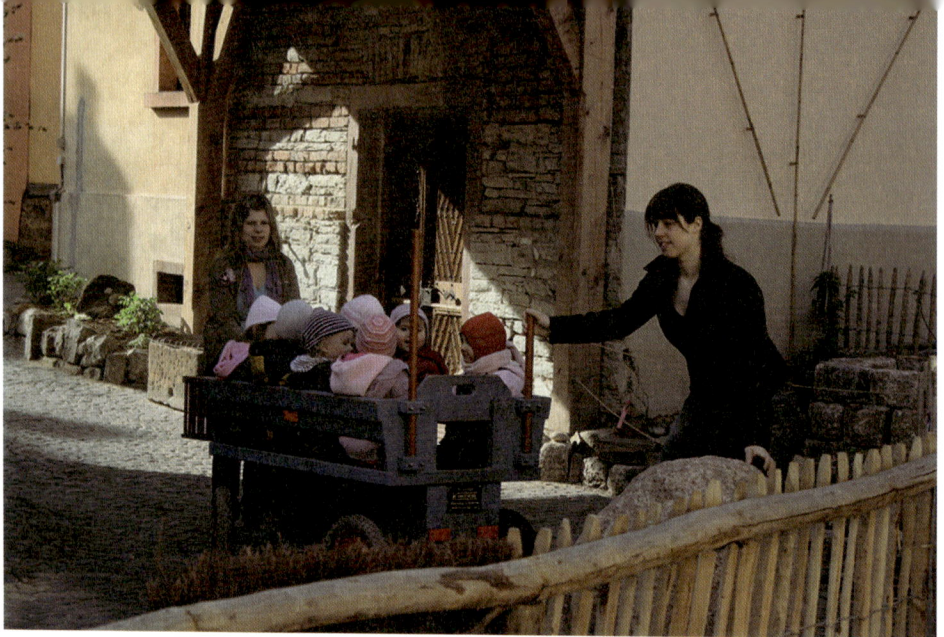

rings of life, the child is embedded in repetitions and rhythms» ... «Time as a circle or a spiral is a calming and healing notion». And further: «Recent research has shown that children can inwardly organize regularly recurring events as early as six months by working out so-called scripts. The script ‹going to sleep› might look like this: Being fed, getting a fresh diaper, being put to bed, falling asleep song, falling asleep.»[1]

For the young child being cared for, there would have to be recurrent «scripts» throughout the day, embedded in a cycle, in a complete script which the child internalizes and in which s/he experiences being protected and feeling secure. In the sense of this inner script forming, he can rely on the repetition.

In this way, the day receives a tangible structure in which reliably one thing follows another. The child also has the security that when a certain period of the caretakers time has been reached, then mother returns. She is included in the script.

The reliability of the daily rhythm is the basis for the little child to be able to engage in the joy of discovery and not to fall into a passive waiting position.

2. The daily rhythm from the point of view of the educators

Caregivers assume a great responsibility, when they decide to look after very young children. The relationship of a mother to her child is emotionally different from the relationship that the caregiver has with the child. The mother and her child are within an accepted mode of mutual dependency. On this basis, the child can also cope with temporary inadequacies that happen with him. Winnicott[2] coined the term «good enough mother». This does not apply to the educator. She has to be «better» than the «good enough educator» in a profes-

---

[1] Michael Schnabel, *Die Vielfalt kindlichen Zeiterlebens*, liga-kind.de/fk-510-schnabel, 5/10, abgerufen 12.4.2018. (the diversity of a child's experience of time)

[2] Vgl. Donald Winnicott, *Transitional objects and transitional phenomena*. In: International Journal of Psychoanalysis, 1953.

sional sense. Accordingly, a «good enough» educator should not exist.

What should be considered?

In the first three years, a child does not only make major developmental steps, but he also establishes his psychic health. The educator must have a comprehensive knowledge about the developmental steps and the emotional needs of the young child, so that she can make sure that the necessary separation from the mother is gentle and does not cause harm, and the child can build new bonds.

On the part of the caregivers, we must ensure that the child is approached with respect for his personality, that s/he is mindfully received and nurtured, carefully accompanied on the path of learning how to eat independently, with sufficient time and space for his free play and discovery, and having his movement-development taking place according to his own pace and self-inspired.

In order to reach professionalism in view of these requirements, we have to learn, practice, and ever again reflect, so that the legitimate claim to be «better» can be fulfilled. The joy in living with the children may not get lost – a relaxed, joyful atmosphere forms the background for a healthy coexistence.

Therefore, the contentment of the children, and the daily rhythm and contentment of the care-givers condition each other. The «institutional reliability» replaces constant agreements and deliberations in between: Who puts diapers on whom, who prepares the foods, what happens next etc. With calm and relaxation, children can be perceived. It is helpful, if every caretaker is informed.

The well-planned daily rhythm, which suits the needs of the child, then also turns out to be helpful and save the strength of the caregivers.

Daily Rhythm as Chart

Time	Daily Rhythm	Children
7:00–8:30	Arrival	free activity
until 8:30	Breakfast when needed right after arrival	free activity
8:30	Care giving if needed	free activity
8:30–9:15	Dressing one after the other, going outside	free activity
beginning at 10:20	Coming inside, first the little ones	free activity
10:30	Lunch: Begin depending on group constellation and age of children	free activity
10:45	Drinking	free activity
10:55	Song, play with hand-gestures together, by choice, some play on	
11:00	Lunch: on lap or on bench or together at the table	free activity
11:35	Caregiving before sleeping	free activity
12:00	One after the other to bed, perhaps some together	
12:00	Nap-time	
14:00	Wake up	free activity
14:30	Tea time, eating	
Approx. 15:00		free activity inside or outside

Adults		
7:00–8:30	Receive children, prepare breakfast, cook lunch.	
8:30	Changing diapers, cleaning up, wash.	
8:30–9:15	Dress children, accompany in play, prepare lunch, clean up.	
From 10:20	Receive children, undress, wash hands, accompany them.	
10:30	Feed lunch, first on lap.	
10:45	Give something to drink.	
11:00	Feed or accompany eating, clean up.	
11:35	Undress, change diapers.	
12:00	Assist going to bed, put on sleeping wear.	
12:00	Clean up, wash dishes, prepare afternoon snack, take turns for a break, documentation.	
14:00	Get children out of bed, change diapers, dress.	
14:30	Accompany tea-time, clean up, wash dishes.	
15:00	Accompany play, make beds, hand over to parents, clean up.	

Claudia Grah-Wittich
To be separate and then together

The little child – as yet an undifferentiated being – is at the mercy of his instincts, is helpless and dependent on the care and protection of the adult. On the other hand, the pedagogical practice shows, that adults have no possibility in the first two to three years to really intervene in the will of the child. The child does, what he wants to do! This contradiction is initially a mystery. But it can become an important starting point for dealing pedagogically with the young child:

How do I support where it is really needed?
How do I further all approaches of his independent and free development?

The child does not need to be actively supported in his or her movement-development nor in play. What he needs, he knows out of himself – as long as he is not disturbed by adults. On the other hand, he brought with him a longing to grow up to be community oriented, and there he is dependent on support by an active relationship-focus. Wherever I enter into active contact with the child, where he needs me, learning about relationship begins.

Of course, this is especially the case with physical care, when eating, changing diapers, wiping nose, dressing and undressing. At first, the child does not do all this out of his own strength, but instead learns from the role model who is actively connecting with him. S/he learns from the other:

- The way the young child is cared for shapes his later social behavior.
- If s/he can develop autonomously and independently in his own movement and in play, it will have an effect on his later sense of responsibility, on his independence, and on his self-confidence in dealing with the world.

Basically, the safer the attachment is to the child, the more self-confident he is in his explorative behavior, his creativity, and his self-sufficient development. And: children want to be noticed in their activity. They seek the gaze of adults and feel encouraged when they are seen.

The power for such creative developing, the child takes from the numerous moments in which he is together with adults and feels well and secure: diapers are put on, he gets to eat, he is comforted, dressed, put to bed – all are activities in which the child is together with us, and we have the heart-warming responsibility to be so with him in such a way, that it gives him pleasure and joy to want to be social, and part of the community.

This always succeeds, when we have time for this togetherness, and when the child has the opportunity to show that he is a naturally co-operative being, who learns more every day: first, the child seems to participate almost imperceptibly when putting on clothes, slowly he helps a bit more, then more and more, until finally the little things and procedures are a matter of course – the child now masters them all by himself. The more we accept the impulses of the child to participate, the sooner he enjoys doing it himself.

The «right» environment is the prerequisite both for the free activity of the child, the self-learning, as well as for the relationship-learning, the being together with the child in the caretaking. Environment is also the attitude, the inner attitude of the adults. When I am, the child can develop.

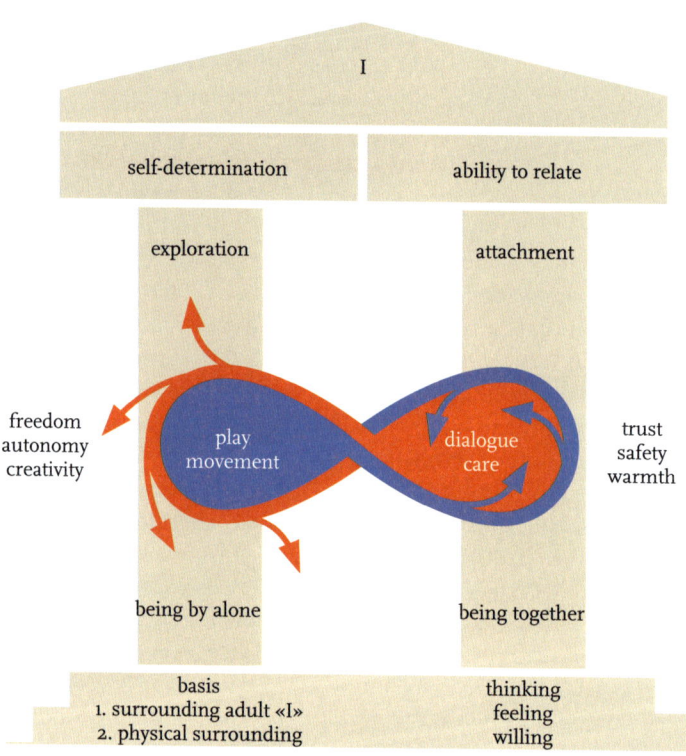

Angelika Knabe
The young child is a being of will

In the fairy tale «Mother Holle» Marie wakes up after she jumps into the well in another world. After some experiences, she comes to the house of Mrs. Holle. She is hard-working there, does everything that she is asked to do, and does it well. Nevertheless, after some time she gets «the misery» and expresses: «I must go back now to my own». She is accompanied by Mrs. Holle a part of the way, and then gets her reward, the golden rain; a new earth life begins.

In the fairy tale, we see that each human being receives his gifts from heaven according to the deeds that they have previously accomplished. These «gift from heaven» are carried along, when s/he begins to start an earthly life again. They have an impact on this new earth life.

But in the beginning there is an impulse of will. Without this cosmic will impulse, we would not be able to begin our new path into incarnation. It is necessary in order to carry out the often arduous and complicated process of the actual incarnation, «the embodiment of the spirit».

Bodily maternal-sheath

We can ask ourselves when the most amazing development on this incarnation path of man is taking place. I think we all agree on that: from egg fertilization to birth. Like a miracle, man evolves completely in secret in his mother's bodily sheaths. The most astonishing development happens in the first three months of pregnancy, when the organism, the tiny physical body, is completely established – after that, the little human only grows and matures.

But even before this human germ comes about, cavities and enveloping boundaries have already formed from the cell tissue. A little later, the developing embryo grows into these.

First, therefore, the environment is formed, the sheath. It is the expression of the inviting gesture of expectation, which should be a basic gesture in infant care.

We should also be aware that in all new stages of development the impulse, the will, always comes from the child. As an example, reference is made to the all-encompassing chorion, the egg-skin, that is to say, the child's tissue, from which villi grow into the maternal tissue. The maternal organism, when it is ready, provides only an answer to the placental formation.

We must clearly visualize the situation of the child in the protective physical sheath of the mother in order to better understand and accompany the developmental processes after birth. On the one hand, the physical maternal cover protects the child from the direct influence of the outer physical world and, on the other, it is the child's first physical environment.

In pregnancy, in this very special time, the mother will take care of herself, but in general she cannot physically directly influence the wonderful process of becoming a human child. This happens *as if by itself*.

To feel at home in the body

... during the earthly life, and only during it, through the use of his body, by plunging into his earthly body, he can experience the impulse of freedom. The human

being can attain freedom only while living on earth, and when entering other worlds, we can take with us only the degree of freedom we have attained here on earth.[1]

Only through the will can the ego immerse itself in his corporeality and become active in his earthly body.

After the birth, in the first year of life, we can recognize this strong incarnational will by how the small infant begins to conquer his body by reducing gradually from head to toe the unconscious reflex movements. From the movement-chaos, the child grasps every movement consciously and purposefully and usually with the utmost concentration. He wants to feel at home in his body and feel good at the same time.

In the directed gaze, the child finds the first stability in the relationship, which now has to be re-gained by the mother and child, that is, from both sides. If the gaze is returned, it develops a strong trust in the child. At the same time, a first delicate differentiation process takes place between here and there. This «Here-am-I»- experience is strengthened in conscious grasping and letting-go-again.

At about nine months, the child overcomes the earth's gravity by virtue of his will and brings his body into the upright, in order to take his first independent steps at about the end of the first year.

This process of taking hold of the body and feeling at home in it, also affects the metabolic organism, albeit largely unconsciously, so that it can work reliably and yet individually.

Through the working of the I in the incarnation-will, – that cannot be imagined without the ego organization, – the child can personally develop the initiative to discover the world more and more in the second year.

By touching, tasting, hearing, seeing, etc., he gets to know the multiplicity of the world. By recalling this variety, by repeatedly pausing, an inner- or personal-space can begin to germinate. Out of this space, his own center, the child can be creative in order to bring his own things into being. Thus, the things of the world are individually recognized and usually named according to their function: The language ability develops.

In the third year, the ego becomes effective and develops ego-consciousness. The first laws in the environment are discovered and investigated. The child can now clearly discern, differentiate, name and remember the world with its details, for the time being without logical reflection.

The Necessity of trust- creating cultural sheaths

In his discoveries, however, the child still needs the security and familiarity of the social home, the security of being protected. When the parents leave, the child quickly starts to show some stranger anxiety and feel very insecure.

I would like to remind you once again of the experience of the lack of protective sheaths that the child feels when, after the

---

[1] Rudolf Steiner, *Soul Economy and Waldorf Education.* Antroposophic Press, GA 303, Lecture 7.

comfort during pregnancy, he has to leave these maternal envelopes which means, the bodily-physical oneness with the mother. The environment of the child suddenly changed very much.

The question now is which environment, which sheaths, and which holding by parents, and later by teachers, is now recreated for the child: «... *what the forces and fluids of the mother's sheath did for it, (the physical body) now, the forces and elements of the external physical world must do*».[2]

Do these new «cultural sheaths» offer the necessary warm and nourishing protection?
Can the child continue to feel at one with his surroundings, so that can he strengthen his physical body, now separated from the mother?
To what extent do we incorporate the forces and elements of the external world into the child's environment?
Can the children still experience something of these beautiful elements of nature in their group rooms?
Or is everything made of dead material, sterile and uniform, flattened and glossed?

Becoming conscious of one-self

As already described above, the child comes into contact with the world through the most diverse sensory perceptions and builds a relationship with the outside world.

---

2 Rudolf Steiner, *The Education of the Child in the Light of Anthroposophy*, GA 34, Rudolf Steiner Press, 1965.

Every sense perception is possible only by the person's willingness to move. Movement, in turn, is an expression of the individual being that wishes to incarnate in this small newly born body.

At the same time, the child becomes more and more aware of himself through the perceptions given by the four body-bound basal senses – but especially through the sense of touch. When practicing, which is always connected with the effort to overcome resistance, and experiencing failures, the child senses joyfully: This is my body, this is me.

Soul sensations express themselves through physical movements – we can read from them whether the child feels joy or grief.

In addition to the experience of his own corporeality, the child becomes more and more aware: I can achieve something with my body. The joy and pride when he experiences – «I can do it»! – is irreplaceable.

In these first seven years of life, but above all in the first three years, the child's main task is to transform the inherited body received from his parents into his own physical tool. Through imitation and sensory impressions his body, his organs are individually imprinted. For this the child needs time, peace, but above all loving care in the widest sense: the right environment.

Lively environment

As the physical mother's sheath surrounds the human being until his/her birth, so s/he is surrounded by an etheric envelope

and an astral envelope until the change of teeth, that is, until the seventh year.[3]
How can we imagine this etheric envelope that surrounds the child until first grade readiness?

We know that the etheric or life body of the newborn child has not yet matured, and is not finished. It is, as during pregnancy the physical body, still dependent on someone else's forces, is still highly in need of protection and therefore dependent on an etheric envelope that surrounds him.

The etheric body develops its own forces first in connection with the inherited foreign forces.[4]

The text quote refers to the etheric envelope created by the closest caregivers of the child. Their attitude and their actions that are influenced by it, are a model for the child and will cause him gradually to imitate these actions willingly. At first it is still a very real «doing-together», a very real co-acting. The child will only be able to imitate when the environment is permeated and shaped by a common will-flow from caregiver and child.

When she looks after the flowers by the window, her will (doing) is directed towards these flowers. This gives the child, usually very close by, the opportunity to be active in the same way, but still for himself. The caregiver penetrates, forms and enlivens with her inner attitude and way of thinking, her and with it the child's closer surroundings.

In what basic mood does the mother or caregiver work?
What relationship does she have to the world?
What habits does she have?

The riddle of the will

How mysterious is the will of the child! If we want to know something about the riddle of the will, we will not influence it from without. If it happens anyway, it acts like an insult, like an attack on the child. This includes the lapidary questions to the child, what it wants to do and what it wants to have. But if we hold back, we can see how the child decides on his/her own what he wants to take in from the variety of things – as if he were reminded of an «instruction» from pre-conceptual times that did not come from a human mouth. For this reason as well, we should treat the childlike will with the utmost respect.

If the adult does the necessary and meaningful work for the common good with the appropriate soul attitude for herself and not for the child, as some kind of a pedagogical measure, then the child can also enjoy his own discoveries in the world in all freedom. The autonomous discovery of the world, in an adult-designed and enlivened environment, is the actual learning for the child.

The differently oriented activities of child and adult can be understood like a common will stream that arises in a roundabout way.

We adults can support this learning through our own enthusiasm by creating the right, inspiring environment. But the child must learn and can only do so on his

---

3 Ibid.
4 Ibid p. 21.

own and will gladly do so, when we accompany him in this process with wakefulness, and comfort him in case of mishaps, and we are really happy about his successes.

Learning spaces instead of teachings and explanations

All teachings, explanations and discussions are disruptive at this age. All decisions that the child is asked to make by himself at this early age have a detrimental effect on his development. Now the objection could come that all thinking and intellectual activity also has an etheric origin. That is true. Teachings and explanations have an effect on the etheric body of the child, which has not yet freed itself at this age. It is only beginning with school readiness that the body-free etheric is in a position to endure the direct action of the intellect: Now the child can learn and think in a new way, with the authority of the teacher supporting the process. An environment prepared by the adult signals to the child that he is allowed to unfold the potentials that he has brought along with him, in the secure and protective presence of the adult.

The child feels overwhelmed only when the environment does not present a completely free offer to participate and imitate: all «educational- and activity- offers», such as, e.g. handcraft instructions are not a learning option for the child at this age, where the child can create out of himself.

Therefore, it cannot be our task to educate children according to a thought-out program, but to provide them with places and spaces where they can experience and learn, where the children can feel comfortable, inspired, and become active.

The most important environment to experience is an upright relationship, the attitude: «Here, we manage together». If the child feels recognized in the togetherness and loved, he is certain that all is «right» the way it is, then he will also not lose the desire to learn. He will unfold and grow beyond himself. More than ever, our children today need the unconditional attention of the adult, who does not take over, does not force the child – perhaps we can also speak here of love ...

Sally Jenkinson
The genius of play

The more intellectual the instruction for young children is already, the more the ideas are dominated by television and video, the more necessary is play and the better we must be able to speak to parents and other educators about the importance and the spirit of play.

Friedrich Froebel said:

Playing is the highest expression of human development in childhood, for only it shows us what is happening in the child's soul. It is the purest and most spiritual product of the child, and at the same time it is a picture of human life on all levels and in all relationships. To the one who has a deeper insight into the human nature, the whole future path of life is revealed in the play freely chosen by the child.[1]

Rudolf Steiner advised us to be attentive to the characteristics of the play activity of each child, especially before the change of teeth during free play.

The individual style, which is noticeable in play until the change of teeth, recurs in some way in the special character of the independent judgment of the human being concerned after the twentieth year of life.[2]

Thus, observing the child's play at home and in the kindergarten can help us gain deep insights into the true nature of the particular human being.

Steiner went on to say how important it is to have an inwardly free soul, an inner being that is not adapted to the world. In our work, we align ourselves with the world and in this way we serve the world; but our souls, he says, must remain free. Our first freedom manifests in our playing, and Steiner emphasizes that if we really believe in an inwardly free soul, then we have to let the children play freely, – anything else would be a sin against the child. Playing is nothing less than the expression of the still unborn spirituality of the child.

A study conducted in British Waldorf kindergartens showed that children played with 54 different themes over a period of eleven days. The observed children loved to play and their play had so much content, «that all of human life could be found in it». This gives us educators a huge challenge:

Can I understand the world of children, stimulate their imagination and give them free space physically and soul-spiritually?
Can I retain a space for them in which their freedom and their spirit can grow and unfold?

Imagination changes reality and imagination is changed by reality – a subtle riddle of the spirit.

The intensity of the memory concerning play, and the power these long-forgotten play-times have over the soul and spirit of the adult is amazing.

In what ways did play help us weave the basic pattern of our individual destiny?

---

1 Friedrich Fröbel, Wichard Lange, *Gesammelte pädagogische Schriften*. Biblio Verlag 1966. (Collected Pedagogical Writings)
2 Rudolf Steiner, *Die Erneuerung der pädagogisch-didaktischen Kunst durch Geisteswissenschaft*. GA 301, Vortrag am 10. Mai 1920 in Basel. Dornach 1986.

Below are excerpts from play stories from around the world:

– **Security:**
I liked to play outside. I knew it was safe because my mother was close by. When she was not there, I could not play as well. She was the necessary foundation for me to feel safe. I did not need to see her, and she did not interrupt my play. Knowing she was there was enough. Often it was more fun to set the rules for a game than to play it. I got to know my surroundings, the landscape, the shortcuts and detours. I learned social behavior; understanding for other children – even for the struggles with the boys.

– **Relationships:**
I remember doing surgery on my bear when I was five or six years old. I had been in the hospital myself at the time. It was a big bear, I cut it open and sewed up again. It was filled with sawdust. I liked cooking and loved «real» play: playing hair-dresser with a proper pair of scissors (and proper trimming!). Relationships were very important to me, both with other children and with teachers. I usually had a «best friend». I loved to play ballerina.

– **Discovery:**
I liked to play alone in the woods. I liked to play with my brother, with the elements, with the earth. In every season I loved being outdoors. Nature was a mysterious world in which I could be alone without fear. I loved the colors, the leaves, the dirt, the feeling of being dry and wet. I always wanted to know: what's behind the next rock?

– **Fantasy:**
I played with my sister dolls and with many other children «king and queen». I loved small berries and big stones. Each stone was a piece of a kingdom, a big stone was a castle. In my imagination there was a beautiful lady and I always hoped she would come to life. For me she was so real that she was actually almost alive.

– **Imitation:**
I lived in a small village in the countryside. My parents had a small grocery store. My little brother and I liked doing all that our parents did. We played shop, but also with the other children in the village.

– **Being by myself:**
We spent the summers at a lake where I was free to develop a strong connection to nature. I loved having plenty of room for myself to be alone with myself.

– **To be active:**
I lived in the countryside, near a bakery, in a small village. I liked baking cakes – with mud and leaves – and we made a complicated oven. I found it fascinating that you could make something and then sell it. Being outdoors in nature was very important to me.

– **Fearlessness:**
I grew up in Texas, in a suburban neighborhood, and had three little brothers. We

played with a neighbor girl in the backyard. The possibilities were very limited, but we still had imaginative adventures when we climbed on the pile of bricks in the yard. We imagined that we were exploring an unknown world. I had a very vivid imagination. Our inner freedom strengthened us. We were fearless; we had dangerous adventures and called ourselves «The Great Girls».

– Transformation:
I loved marbles because of their beautiful colors. The swirling patterns in the marbles had a special magic for me. We became more and more skilled and collected the marbles that we won in a large jar. I was the oldest of four children and had two sisters and one brother. We dressed up as princes and princesses and spread out a carpet to march over in procession. I particularly remember this ability of transformation, and I remember colors – light and colors.

Chart for the children's play
Children play best,
- if adults pay attention, but do not interfere; when the feeling of safety encourages discovery and adventure in the children;
- if the trust in life remains in tact for children, so that they are open and fearless in face of the unknown;
- if they have space in the world; if there is enough free space to conquer for themselves;
- if adults have no expectations of their play, if no «final» result is asked for;
- when their senses are directly inspired by nature and the elements;
- when they have freedom, time and opportunity, to become collectors, manufacturers and world creators;
- if they can play with other children and socialize; if they can also be alone and completely undisturbed by themselves;
- if in their play with others and in their own imagination they are able to develop self-assurance;
- if they can communicate themselves, their joy, their grief and their worries without fear of being laughed at or not taken seriously; if mystery and imagination are not paralyzed by so-called facts;
- when playing is recognized as the central activity in the life of a child.

This charter shows just how valuable play is for the child and the central role it plays in childhood. Play prepares the development of freedom and enables the fulfillment of not yet manifest karmic-spiritual aspirations. A child who cannot play freely will have difficulties later in life with independence. Educators who assume that children develop independence if they are increasingly equipped with academic skills, are on a false path. Intuition through play should come before instruction. In the lecture given by Rudolf Steiner in Nürnberg, on November 14, 1910, he said that we should avoid any standardization in education, but especially in play-activity. Play must be something individual, and we should pay attention to the talents and interests of each individual child. If we do not, he said, we would sin against the child. On January 12, 1911, he says in Berlin:

Through play-activity we work back in a free, definable way on the soul-spiritual organization of the human being. Play and the just characterized soul-spiritual activity of the child in the first years rise out of a deep awareness of what the nature and being of the child actual is.[3]

Tina Bruce, the English Early Childhood Education expert[4], recommends to follow the play of the individual children and to pay particular attention to the patterns chosen, such as «wrapping», «enclosing», «throwing», etc. She assumes that certain subjects and forms repeat themselves and that a child works with a kind of muse for a certain time and then goes on to something else. The same forms show themselves, she goes on to show, for example, when building with wooden blocks on the floor, when baking bread, in movement games and when drawing. Piaget[5] also recognized the importance of the play and saw imitation as a force that stimulates learning and emotional life.

Conditions for free play

Playing is often too short in our kindergartens and is not always really free.

What makes free play possible?

Children must have the opportunity to develop three different spheres while playing:
- the cultural-social sphere (puppetry, theatre performances);
- the political-legal sphere (territory, tribal affiliation, war games);
- the economic sphere (grocery store, dealer).

Because in play the history of humankind is mirrored.

Adults busily working are particularly stimulating for playing children.

However, interfering or playing along should be avoided. Adults need to be courageous and tolerant about safety precautions. They should not intervene too early in a squabble, as children are often able to transform situations themselves.

Children must have the opportunity to challenge themselves in their play. «Toys» do not seem to be as valuable as just «stuff». The value is more in being occupied than in beauty.

As long as goodness, beauty and truth in the inner environment (adults) are not neglected, everything is alright that can appeal to the imagination. Often, the things we want to throw away provide the biggest incentive to play.

Children need time to play, even outdoors, in any season.

Young children need even more space and time to play.

---

[3] Rudolf Steiner, *Antworten der Geisteswissenschaft auf die großen Fragen des Daseins*. GA 60, Vortrag am 12. Januar 1911 in Berlin. Dornach 1983. *(The Answers of Spiritual Science to the Big Questions of Existence)*

[4] Tina Bruce, *Learning Through Play: For Babies, Toddlers and Young Children*.

[5] Jean Piaget, * 9. August 1896 in Neuchâtel; † 16. September 1980 in Geneva, was a Swiss developmental psychologist und Epistemologist. He developed genetic epistemology. Piaget believes that people are open systems, that strive for constant balance and seek equilibrium. The organism strives for knowledge, or has a need for knowledge about what is important for it. Being becomes active through this drive, the open system develops. (Wikipedia)

Pictures from stories help play, they are flexible and let the soul breathe.

Adults need to develop a listening sense, for when the child's play is healthy and when not.

Children like to play where they are not seen.

Claudia Grah-Wittich
Play-levels[1]

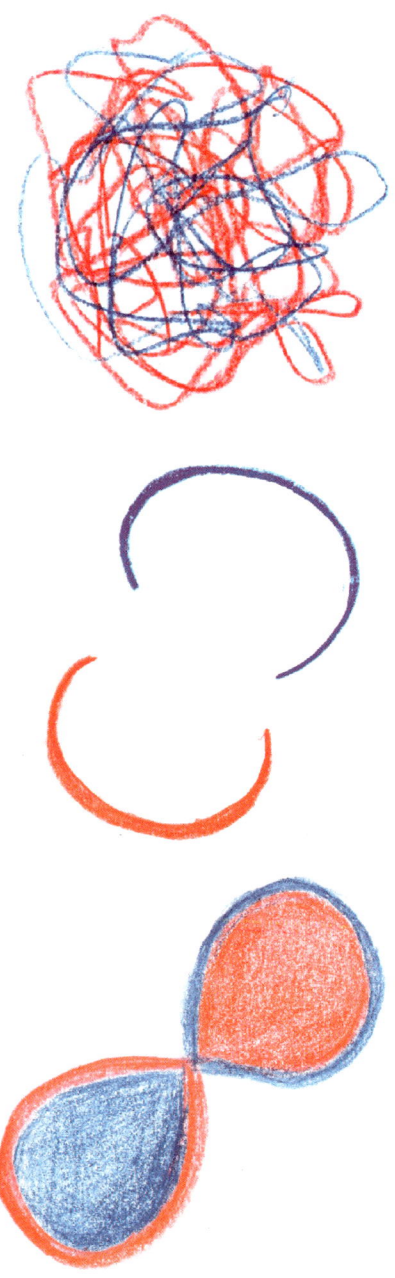

The child comes into the room and is not yet oriented. S/he seeks nothing definite, does not pursue any intention. She listens to the atmosphere in the room, is receptive for everything, that comes from the outside. She is open to being attracted by one thing, and that this attraction will lead to an impulse. Warmth determines whether something will develop out of one's own impulse – with her behavior the child mirrors her environment.

The child finds something to do, still seemingly random, out of the abundance of possibilities. Something arouses her attention. The toys still remain as if outside of her, although she takes them into her hand, tries them, and looks for play-variations. The familiar processes are repeated. She tries to get a picture of what is (around). Now it is important for a child to find suitable, age-appropriate possibilities for movement and play: and whether she can discover herself through them. By discovering things, she discovers herself in space.

The child dives completely into her playing, loses herself in the environment. If we would talk to her, she would not hear us. The world is lost, child and world are one (this concerns play *and* movement). This process repeats itself, turns rhythmic and pulsates. In this deep connecting new experiences can be integrated and digested. We can speak here of a phase of appro-

---

[1] Entwicklungsstufen in Anlehnung an die Entwicklungsstufen der Erde. In: Rudolf Steiner, *Die Geheimwissenschaft im Umriss*. GA 13.

priation of abilities, whereby a living stream flows between the child and the environment: The object-world becomes alive and can be processed internally. This is where the prerequisites for self-learning are created. Concentration, joy and repetition characterize the crossing point of the encounter. The child experiences self-efficacy at this interface. The ego experience is initiated.

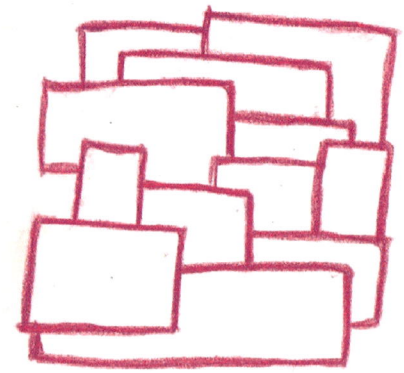

The child completes a variation of her play. She does not make any new experiences, but processes the experience gained. Before she starts a new variation, she seeks rest and recovery, and enjoys them. From this resting, an echo lingers on. A new impulse can come.

The levels of play, but also all other stages of development, always follow the same laws. In today's fast paced world, we can notice that children often cannot move from the second level to the third, because of the variety of programs offered. We then speak of «restless children». However, if we do not disturb children in their play from the beginning, they will develop themselves in the above-described rhythm.

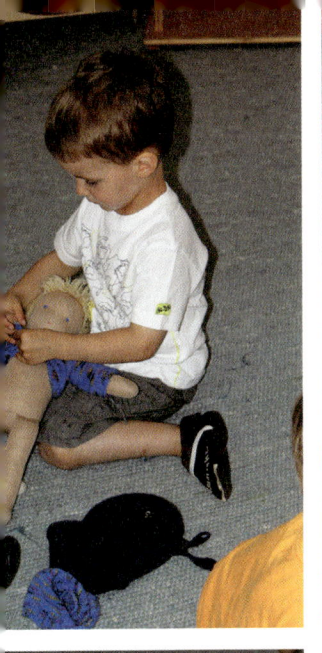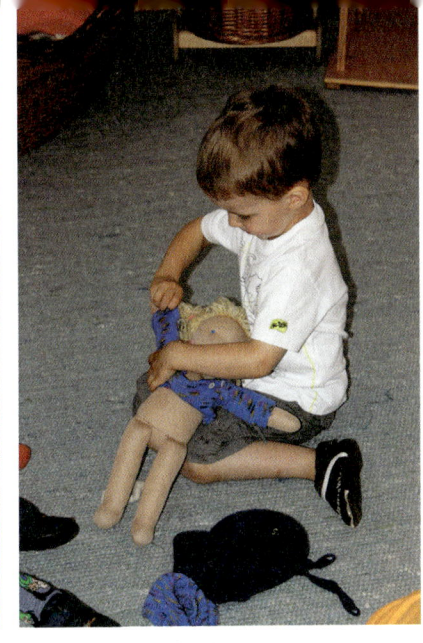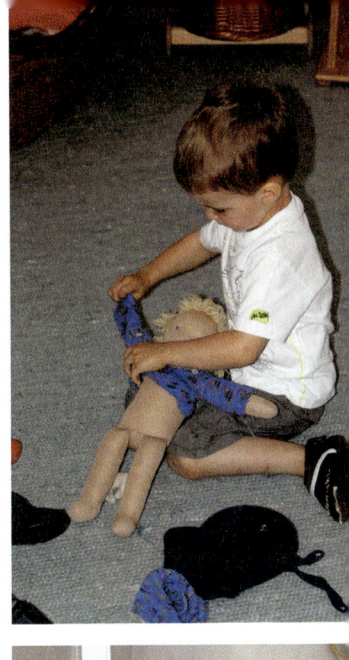
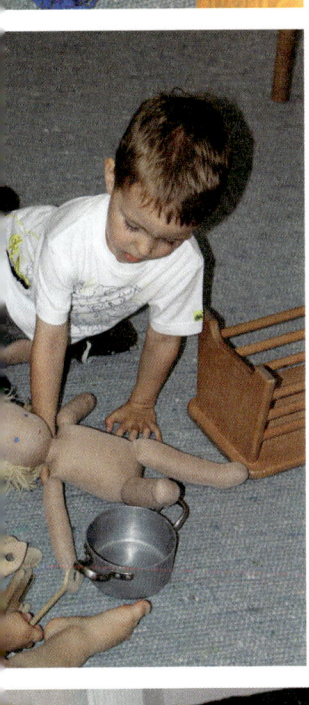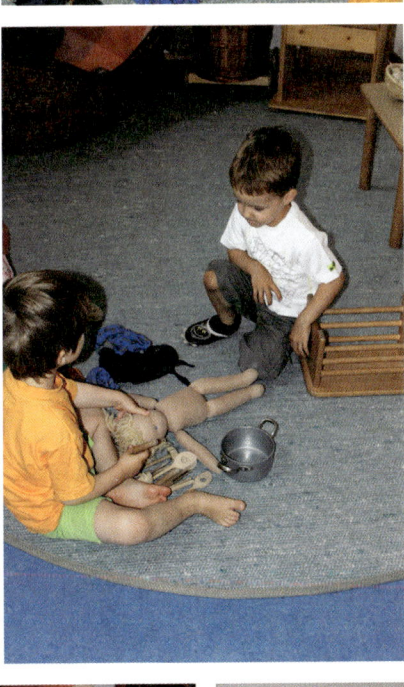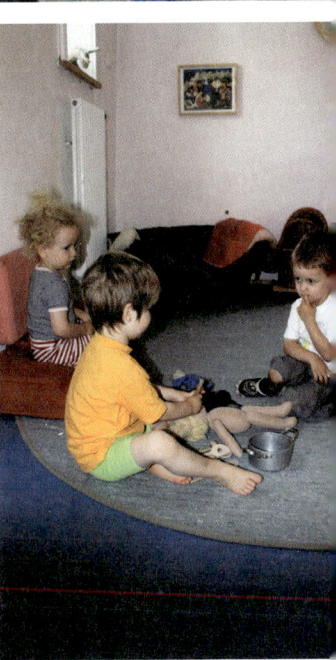
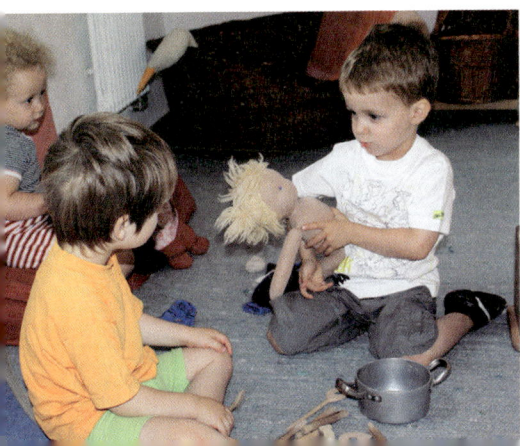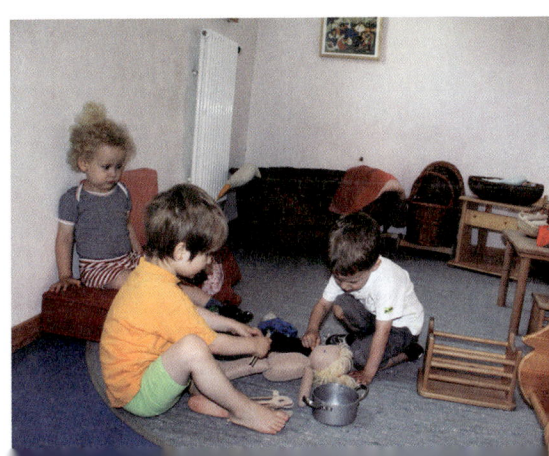

Rolf and Inge Heine

Caring is education – education is caring

When does education begin?

This is a question asked by researchers, teachers and primarily of course by parents expecting a child. Rudolf Steiner's insightful answer is:

The less one thinks about educating the child before it even sees the light of day and the more one focuses on leading one's own life in the right way, the better will it be for the child.[1]

Thus whoever wishes to educate a child with music will certainly achieve far more by singing, making or listening to music during pregnancy than by playing a CD through the abdomen to the foetus.

Care of the new born infant and young child

The child in the womb is fully provided for by the maternal organism and the awareness of the mother. This changes radically at birth: The child leaves the protective, warm and nourishing sheaths that have surrounded it for nine months in a weightless, fluid environment. With its first breath it connects with the world outside; with its umbilical chord cut it must now form a completely new relationship to its surroundings as an independent organism. It must learn to breathe, to regulate its own body temperature, digest its food, to synchronize its rhythm of sleeping and waking with its food intake, the light and its social context, it must come to terms with gravity and much else besides. This huge process of adaptation is supported by reflexes (breathing, movement) and instincts (such as hunger and suckling) but it also requires the ongoing help of the mother or another care person – the child needs to be kept clean, fed, carried, protected, given a rhythm, warmed and brought into balance if it is to survive.

It is however not only these more bodily aspects of the child that caring for. In order to learn the specifically human capacities – upright walking, speaking and thinking – the child needs the example of adults. Walking, speaking and thinking cannot be developed without an example. Neither can a stable, open-minded attitude of soul.

It will be determined mainly by the surroundings, an in particular through the emotional attachment to the main care person. Potential creativity, artistic ability and behavior are likewise encouraged or hindered by the person the child relates to.

We can therefore distinguish two areas the child requires help with:
1. Physical care to help the child's organism adjust to its surroundings.
2. Development of the specifically human qualities and care for the child's soul space.

The second area belongs in the narrower sense to education, the first to (physical) care. During the first three years both care and education are essentially focused on the physical body. Care and education are as yet indistinguishable from one another. To separate care into a physically «essential» part (nappy changing, washing) and a behavioral program (word play, cuddling, playing) makes no sense when we consider that it is through the loving attention to

---

[1] Rudolf Steiner, *The Study of Man*. GA 293, Lecture 1.

physical needs that the child learns to trust, find security, direct its movements, learn meaningful sequences of movement as well as explore the most varied objects and materials. Apart from this it is now known that the first step towards acquiring speech or behavioral patterns comes through the imitation of movements (facial muscles, copying, the hands, gesture etc.).

In what follows a description will be given of how through care the foundation is laid for developing the child's soul-spiritual and social capacities. The various aspects of caring will be classified according to the twelve gestures of nursing[2]. They indicate how the attitude of the care person or educator is made visible through the way in which daily care activities are carried out. The term «gesture» indicates that in each nursing activity a quality is expressed that goes beyond the immediate sense perceptible effect of the care and touches on the totality of the human being in body, soul and spirit.

The 12 care gestures as care and education in harmony

The following sequence – new-born infant – toddler – kindergarten child – refers to the stages in child development rather than a specific age. With the term new-born infant we mean the age of approximate 0–6 months, with toddler 6 months to 3 years, with kindergarten child 3–6 year.

Cleansing

The gesture of cleansing	Focus is directed towards that innocent being which is dirty. What is old and impure is carefully removed. The washed body then appears as new. The hand of the care person removes the old in order to allow the new to emerge. A joyous feeling of expectation towards what wishes to appear. Matter-of-fact interest and sober objectivity towards what needs disposing. The action should be careful, well-managed, quick and deliberate.
Examples of cleansing with the new-born infant	When the child is born amniotic fluids and slime are removed from the air passages, secretions are mopped up, Meconium, urine, umbilical residues etc. are disposed of.
with the toddler	Faeces, urine, sweat, food remnants, dirt etc. are removed. The child is washed, bathed, nails are cut and teeth are brushed.

---

2 Rolf Heine, *Das Konzept der Zwölf pflegerischen Gesten*. In: De la Houssaye, E., *Beiträge zur Entwicklung der Anthroposophischen Pflege*. Dornach 2005.

with the kindergarten child	The kindergarten child is increasingly able to wash itself independently. Some aspects such as for example the brushing of teeth, should continue to be monitored by an adult. The child grows adept when its independence is encouraged. This means that sufficient time should be allowed for each individual step in the washing procedure. Kindergarten children like trying to wash each other or their dolls. The social aspects of care are then imitated.
What must be taken into account with cleansing?	Cleansing should take place on a well prepared nappy table. The height of the table should be such as to be kind to the back and facilitate communication with the child. Sides give protection and prevent the child from rolling of the table. The mother, father or nurse announces each step of the process with gentle words. Their gestures give the same message as the spoken words. The child is only turned on its side, its legs are not lifted upwards. The turning on its side corresponds to the natural development of movement and prepares the child for the time when at about half a year old, it is able to turn itself on to its side.
What does the child «learn» when being washed?	Giving a name to the actions, correlating word and deed, encourages the development of speech. The gestures and mimicry of the child mirror the gestures and mimicry of the adult caring for it and are an immediate expression of pleasant or unpleasant feelings. The development of movement is encouraged through the child experiencing the dimensions of space on its own body. More advanced stages of development should not imposed upon it ahead of time (no passive sitting before the child has learnt to sit up by itself; no standing before it has learnt to pull itself upright). Washing and care of the body is practiced as a form of social interaction and becomes an example of self care and the care of others.
Feeding	
Feeding as a gesture	The person feeding needs to experience joy in making a gift and having respect for the food. He must know how difficult it is for the child to take in and incorporate the food. Parents need to be patient with the processes of digestion. «Love goes via the stomach». «The human being does not live by bread alone».
Examples of feeding new-born infants	The appropriate form of nourishment for the new-born infant is breast milk. With breast feeding it is not only about physical nourishment (breast milk with its optimal make up for each stage of development) but also about the time given to the child, the peace, the bodily closeness and devotion. These are all woven into the mother's milk. With breast feeding cosmic (soul-spiritual) nutrition and earthly (bodily) nutrition are still one indivisible whole. Breast feeding is one of the most important factors in the bonding of mother and child.

toddlers	After 6 months the period of breast feeding is gradually supplemented with other forms of nutrition. The variable rhythm of breast feeding is now replaced by an introduced rhythm. Food is given first on the lap and then more independent eating is encouraged in a high chair. The mother's preparation for breast feeding now becomes the preparation of food and the meal that is to be given on the lap and later in the high chair. The close connection of the breast feeding mother is now broadened out through certain rituals (washing of hands, table grace, feeding and then providing assistance with eating as it becomes more independent and blessing the meal). Food for the body and food for soul now begin to separate. Until the child is able to eat entirely on its own, the 1:1 care relationship remains in place.
with the kindergarten child	The kindergarten child is now able to eat so independently that it can participate in the family meal times. It needs help with regard to the choice, amount and mixture of the food. While eating in the high chair still formed part of a more limited mother-child relationship, sitting together as a family for a meal, becomes an important social event. The food is shared. Patience and mutual respect must be balanced against the drive to satisfy hunger and thirst. The tastes of the various foods awaken feelings of sympathy or antipathy. The child can already help to prepare the food, can have tasters and help to lay the table.
What should be observed with feeding?	All impatience should be avoided when feeding and when eating food in general. Soul-spiritual needs (for closeness, dedication, comfort) should not be compensated for by giving food or addictive substances (sweets). High quality food (e.g. grown biodynamically) is rich in taste and flavor and needs no additives.
What does the child «learn» when it is fed?	The child trains its sense of life between the poles of hunger and the feeling of being satisfied. Beyond this it experiences the interaction between bodily and social rhythms. It experiences that the world is good. It experiences peace through the satisfaction and gratitude for having received the «gift» of food. Through eating together, it develops the ability to share, to say what it wants and to balance it against the needs of others. Table manners should therefore be taught by the parents' example and not through disciplinary measures. Only in this way can the ritual of eating together engender gratitude and the creation of a religious mood. Helping with cooking and cooking for the dolls, sharing out and gifting – these are important steps in the training of social competences.

Supporting, letting go, helping

Letting go as a gesture	The all-round vulnerability of the child calls forth on the part of adults a deep-seated urge to provide help. It is first necessary however to identify the areas of need. They are found on the physical, soul and spiritual levels. This calls upon the care person's sense for what is helpful. The gesture of wanting to help permeates all care activities and should be filled with a heart-felt and joyful willingness to serve the child. All of its needs must be taken seriously. The actions of the one helping are experienced as selfless and self-evident. It is about being able to carry warmth and light in the heart and providing the child with what it needs.
Examples of letting go with regard to the new-born infant	Without the help of an adult the new-born infant could not survive. The adult ensures its needs are met. Thanks to this help the child is able develop in both body and soul. The child's dependency on the adult becomes particularly noticeable when its position is changed. In the womb the child is always with the mother. After its is born there are quite naturally periods of spatial separation. The new-born infant needs to be held and carried by the adult. In being carried both gravity and this feeling of separation is overcome.
with the toddler	The toddler is continuously progressing with its movement. Quite independently it gradually learns to crawl, sit, stand and walk. As its capacity to move increases, dependency on the adult grows less and its movement radius widens. In order to ensure that the (movement) intentions of the child do not run counter to those of the adult, a safe space reflecting its current ability must be created where the child can freely follow its impulse to move, experience itself and meet the world. The gesture of – helping, carrying, letting go – recedes in favor of the gesture of warding off danger.
with the kindergarten child	The kindergarten child becomes increasingly able to carry out daily care activities (washing, getting dressed, walking, carrying ...) in a focused and goal orientated way. All such activity is a form of serious play and must arise out of the child's own impulses. The adult encourages the attainment of such goals by being aware of the effort the child is making. The child should not be corrected, criticized or diverted. Expecting too much is just as damaging as not having trust in its ability.
What should be considered with regard to carrying or releasing?	There is a danger of paralyzing a child's autonomy and keeping it in dependency by being over protective. Impulses for greater autonomy are easily overlooked.

What does the child «learn» when it is helped?	The child experiences through being carried (and through all kinds of support) that its own impulses can be encouraged and brought to fruition through others. It learns to ask for and accept help and to cooperate. Being dependent on help means the child encounters the theme of «power and powerlessness». The fundamentals of social life are thereby addressed and prepared – throughout our lives we depend on the support of other people. I must adjust my own wishes and intentions to those of others. I learn to cooperate, to insist or to comply.

Protecting

Protecting as a gesture	Protecting against danger means that awareness is focused wholly towards the outside. The one being protected is in the centre, the care person turns her back to the child and creates a boundary by focusing on its surroundings. The care person then has no direct connection to the child – he is preoccupied with the «defence operation». This gesture is often taken up by the father as a means of ensuring that the child is not prematurely confronted with the world outside.
Examples of protecting a new-born infant	The new-born infant has lost the protection of its mother's body. It is presented with a huge number of rapidly changing sense impressions. It cannot remove itself from them. They have a deep effect on its bodily organism. Apart from guarding it against the more obvious environmental threats (getting cold, over heating, suffocation, infection ...) the protection against excessive sense impressions (noise, careless handling, bright light, changing persons to relate to, stress ...) are also important tasks of the educator.
a toddler	When the child broadens its movement horizon, the sources of potential danger in the environment need to be made safe (plug sockets, insecure furniture, things that can be swallowed, electrical equipment ...). The basic principle is to arrange the surroundings in such a way that there is no need to prevent the child from doing something, that a realm is created where the child is able to move safely.
a kindergarten child	The kindergarten child gradually learns to deal with potential sources of danger – to recognize and avoid them. The old «protective barriers» can be gradually removed in order to give space to the child's inquisitive spirit. Protection against over-strong sense impressions, an excessive amount of activity and against new dangers, must continue to be practiced.

What should be considered with regard to protecting?	When focusing on protection there is a danger of being preoccupied with threats and forgetting about the forces of resistance and self-healing potential that are present in every person. It is also harmful, if in the zeal for safety the one in need of protection is forgotten. Whoever seeks to prevent it coming into contact with what is harmful, isolates the child and denies it the opportunity of learning how to deal with danger. A further problem with this approach is that by transferring one's own anxieties, the child is made more insecure and therefore more dependent.
What does the child «learn» when it is protected?	The child can feel secure and safe in a protected space. It experiences that «the world is good». It is open for new experiences – and can learn to overcome the limitations.

Arranging space, creating order

Ordering as a gesture	Meaningful order comes about between chaos and a rigid structure. In bringing about order awareness oscillates between the child and its surroundings and the space between centre and periphery is given a structure – everything has its place and is returned to its place afterwards. Order is the harmonious relationship between the part and the whole. Order in time brings about rhythm.
Examples of bringing about order with new-born infants	During pregnancy space is created for the child within the mother's body. The outer surroundings must also be prepared for the child. When the child is born the course of the day needs to be restructured. It must be adapted on the one hand to the needs of the child and on the other to the requirements of the wider social context. The healthy new-born infant is seeking a rhythm for itself between feeding and digesting, between sleeping and waking, between being alone and being with its mother. The adults need to adjust to these rhythms and bring the surrounding conditions into harmony with them.
with the toddler	With the toddler a certain amount of temporal and spatial structure has established itself. The adults remain responsible for maintaining order or continually re-establishing it in the form of the day's rhythmic structure and keeping order in the play room.
with the kindergarten child	The kindergarten child can adapt itself to appropriate social rhythms such as common meal times, sleeping times, play periods and rest hours. It needs to have clear spatial order. It knows the places where things are kept. It enjoys ordering things in a playful way and then dissolving the order once again. It is however not able to maintain spatial or temporal order independently. That remains the responsibility of the adults. The child loves to take part in bringing about order in a playful way especially when it experiences the joy that adults have in it.

What must be considered in relation to order?	Order does not come about by itself. It requires considerable creative power. Pedantic order, inflexible planning and rigid concepts should be avoided.
What does the child «learn» when it is able to live in an ordered environment?	Order makes it possible for the child to experience familiarity, security and clarity. Good habits are encouraged. The child finds its place and feels well received and wanted. Living rhythms and order provide a source of well being and awaken in the child a sense for what is beautiful, for what is proportional and adequate. The living creation by adults of spatial order and a rhythmic life acts like a «pre-school» for developing the child's musical and mathematical skills.

Surrounding

Surrounding as a gesture	This gesture comes right from the centre. It generally comes about through great sympathy. The care person becomes aware of his own surroundings and clothes the child in them. The strength for doing this comes from the care person's own connection to the surroundings. By creating this surrounding of warmth a space is created in which the forces of growth and development can work. It is the pre-condition for enabling the organs to mature, for regeneration and growth.
Examples of surrounding with the new-born infant	The unborn child grows within an all encompassing and surrounding sheath. It is due to this surrounding (yolk sack, the mother's womb ...) that its entire development occurs. Shortly after it is born the child is wrapped in cloths. The close bodily contact with the mother forms a new sheath. Cloth and clothing surround the new-born infant in the same way as warm concern and care should also do.
with the toddler	With every stage in its development the child sheds another cloak. It leaves first its mother's body, then the confines of the cradle – it is perhaps placed in a cot. In learning to walk, speak and think it emancipates itself ever further from the primal «nest». The more secure its connection has been to the first main care person, the easier will it be for the child to have trust in new connections. So long as it has not yet developed its own physical and social sheaths (up to 21!) and depending on its stage of development, it will need warmth, affection and clothing.
with the kindergarten child	The kindergarten child leaves the protection of its previous surroundings and focus person(s) and enters new social situations. In the first year of its life the child learns skills in «self care». It learns increasingly to care for its own surroundings, to wash itself, get dressed. It playfully cares for, washes, combs and dresses dolls; together with others it dresses up and surrounds itself with cloth and play clothes.

What needs considering with surrounding?	These surrounding sheaths create a warm and structured inner space. They must however not be too tight. The gesture of creating a protective surrounding is generally inspired by sympathy and there is a danger of over protecting, of suffocating, of crushing the child, of creating a mutually dependent symbiosis or of even finding pleasure in the child's dependency. Clarity and sober thinking helps guard against over protectiveness.
What does the child «learn» when it is surrounded?	The child matures in the physical surroundings of its body and in the social fabric of family, crèche and kindergarten. It experiences how it is surrounded by the warmth, air, food and limitations of a secure and positive living space. The security of relationship with its mother or another primary care figure, allows it to expand its horizons and makes its own connections (surroundings). Only a person who is thus surrounded (loved) is able to surround (love) another.

Balancing

Balancing as a gesture	Here it is about balancing out one-sided qualities and producing a dynamic centre – where there is too much, to reduce it, where there is too little to add something. This gesture contains the approach needed for teasing out the appropriate gesture of care – a one-sided quality is recreated and inwardly enhanced to the point where the necessary counter movement becomes conscious. Mutual feeling – empathy – is the means of perception. The gesture appears as an internal «complementary after image».
Examples of creating balance with the new-born infant	Immediately after it is born the new-born infant has to adapt itself to completely new conditions in its surroundings. It is able neither to regulate its own body temperature, move in any directed way nor control its excretions. Through the care they give, the adults balance out what is missing or is there in excess (stilling hunger, giving warmth, carrying, cleansing …).
with the toddler	Although the toddler is able to express its needs more clearly than the new-born infant, it is still not able on its own to provide the necessary balance. The utterances and intentions of the child need to be acknowledged, responded to and if necessary brought into balance by the adults.
with the kindergarten child	The capacities for self-regulation in the kindergarten child are also far from being fully developed. It is however increasingly able to participate actively in the relevant balance inducing activities. Forms of play that develop balance (climbing, balancing) are greatly enjoyed.

What must be considered with regard to balance?	Balance brings about a reduction in tension. Needs and tensions, must, can and should also be borne to a certain degree. If adults are unable to cope with extremes (e.g., high fever) they can more readily control their own needs than children. Static, conceptually determined averages or the falling from one extreme into the other, should be avoided.
What does the child «learn» through balance?	With stable and balanced parents or educators the child is able to experience the capacity for wakeful inner mobility. It learns to trust in the fact that no extreme situation, no sorrow and also no joy, can last forever.

Stimulating

Stimulating as a gesture	A stimulus follows an intention. The stimulus often occurs as a result of a directed, time limited and spatially localized movement or contact designed to call forth a certain reaction. An external stimulus provokes an inner reaction. «Friction produces warmth». Giving direct stimulation requires one to have wakeful and exact observation, focused and measured action and an ability to wait patiently and expectantly.
Examples of stimulating with regard to the new-born infant	Breathing, circulation, the taking in of food, even the excretions of the new-born infant receive a strong stimulus through having direct bodily contact with the mother (breast feeding, bonding). This direct bodily contact is gradually replaced by the bodily care, by the dressing, playing, stroking or massaging.
with the toddler	In the case of the toddler the experience of nature is added to the stimuli of body and soul. Walking in the woods, meadows and fields allows a meeting with wind and weather, with sun, light and shadow. Encounters with other children including in the context of nursery school, has a particularly stimulating effect on body and soul.
with the kindergarten child	The discovery of the plant, animal and mineral kingdoms stimulates the development of imagination, speech and thinking ability in the child. Further, secure fields of activity are required in order to give full reign to its inquisitive interest. Fairy tales give imaginative expression to the experience of nature and of human relationships. In this way they have a stimulating effect on the child's moral development. In the case of illness the use of poultices and compresses or oilings support the self-healing forces. Compresses (for example a chamomile oil tummy compress) allows the child to be wrapped around and attended to like a «baby» once again. This «therapeutic regression» stimulates the forces of growth in body and soul. Most children enjoy this treatment.

What must be considered with stimulation?	Stimulation can also quickly lead to sensory overload especially when parents or educators become impatient. The effect of a particular gesture always depends on the dosage used. *Life is full of stimulation. Stimulation in its turn is something to be used with caution – it should be neither too powerful nor too weak. Weak stimuli help to form organs, medium strong ones strengthen them, very strong ones inhibit and excessive stimuli destroy.*[3]
What does the child «learn» through stimulation?	A child that receives direct encouragement and stimulation can understand the world as a field for learning and experience, or even as a medicine. It learns to develop a certain «therapeutic feeling» which may be expressed through the way it acts or later on engages in its vocation.

Hindering

Hindering as a gesture	In meeting a hindrance the child is challenged to do something which it is able to achieve through own resources. The child has the capacity for instance to develop its own movements. It is expected to experience little disappointments too in the knowledge that what lives as a need will find satisfaction elsewhere or that an effort (for example trying grasp a ball) will eventually bring success.
Examples of hindering in a new-born infant	Living into its new environment presents existential challenges (responsibility) for the new-born infant. Despite the support of its parents (gesture of letting go) it will not be possible to free the child of all its burdens or protect it entirely from its confrontation with the environment. The main carer should observe where and how the child takes its own initiative to solve a problem or overcome some resistance. In principle, every requirement is a burden. The searching and sucking movements of the infant shows that the child wishes to drink – they represent such an «initiative» which the mother should then respond to through the gesture of «feeding».
with the toddler	From the perspective of adults the toddler is exposed to continual frustrations. Its ability to move forward and its fine motor skills are often not sufficient for it to reach its target. At the same time, we can observe the tremendous will power that is repeatedly applied, to overcome this «failure» until gradually, it becomes more skilful and certain in its movements, in walking and speaking. The joyful (sometimes also impatient) efforts of the child should not be subverted by premature «aids».

---

3 Hugo Kükelhaus, in: http://www.hugo-kuekelhaus.eu/.

with the kindergarten child	The older the child becomes, the greater are the expectations of adults regarding certain skills and achievements. Parents compare the «abilities» of their own children with those of others and worry if their own child is not yet walking, not yet potty trained, still not speaking whole sentences, cannot dress alone, doesn't sleep through the night … Justified concern about the child's health is often overlaid with ideas projected from the adult world about targets and achievement. That is why «Give me time»[4] is the most important maxim for early childhood education. The placing of excessive demands on achievements that are inappropriate to a child while simultaneously curtailing the child's activity because it is «clumsy» and «would take too long» or demanding unnecessary rules of behavior (for example insisting on holding hands in situations where there is no danger), is something that often occurs on a daily basis to the kindergarten child.
What should be considered with regard to hindering?	It is unnecessary to create hindrances, training programs or plan exercises unless they are needed therapeutically to balance out one-sided qualities that have been inherited or accrued. During the course of its socialization process the healthy child will «of itself» usually be confronted by such challenges. From this perspective health may be defined as the ability to develop the forces necessary to overcome hindrances and resistance.
What does the child «learn» through hindering?	The child gains strength by meeting age-appropriate obstacles. Through them its will is strengthened. Disappointment and frustration on the other hand caused by being continually over burdened, weakens self confidence and even affects the immune system. Low expectations and the avoidance of hindrances that can be overcome, weaken the will.

Waking up

Waking up as a gesture	The process of waking up accompanies and mediates the journey from the unconsciousness of sleep into a conscious awareness of the world and oneself. It is the path from the «darkness of the body» to the «light of the senses» and later to the «world of thinking». The awakening child should, step by step, gradually find itself.

---

4 Emmi Pikler, *Laßt mir Zeit! (give me time!)* 3rd edition. München 2001, p. 178.

Examples of waking up with the new-born infant	The new-born infant sleeps for more than two thirds of the day. When it is awake, countless sense impressions are absorbed which it can neither consciously process (understand) nor react directly to. Sense impressions therefore have a strong effect on the body. The new-born infant should be kept as far as possible, in familiar surroundings close to its mother (or its main carer). Sense impressions coming through ear and eye should not be too strong; everything that is stressful, glaring, loud, brash, must be avoided. According to Rudolf Steiner: «*Mother's milk has an awakening effect on the slumbering human spirit*»[5].
with the toddler	The toddler is increasingly open to receive sense impressions. It would like to find out where they come from but also keep them at a distance. Everyday objects and toys which are simply constructed and are transparent and stimulating for a broad spectrum of sensory experience, can be readily recognized and be more deeply understood.
with the kindergarten child	With the first glimmerings of ego consciousness the ability to distinguish between the connections to mother, father, siblings, relatives or other people in the vicinity, begins to awaken. The child starts to become aware of its social surroundings. Play acting and dressing up broaden the scope of play.
What should be considered with regard to waking up?	The important thing about awakening is that the one who acts as «awakener» is able to identify intensively with the child's state of consciousness. Only then can he develop the necessary circumspection and patience for leading it towards the world of sense impressions. Every lighting up of consciousness, (for instance a smile, a look, in the first sounds and words) is a source of joy. Sensory overload and the premature awakening of the intellect should be avoided. Imaginative stories and immersion in color and form encourages a gradual awakening towards the world.
What does the child «learn»?	The child experiences the joy of discovery and of knowledge; it experiences an inner light, the discovery of itself.
Affirming	
Affirming as a gesture	Parents or educators need to be sure that whatever they are doing is meaningful. This gives the action a quality of optimism and hope for the future. The past is looked at positively and from the perspective of transformation. One has an experience of inner balance. Faithfulness, empathy and an optimistic attitude towards life and destiny, make up this gesture.

---

[5] Rudolf Steiner, *The Study of Man.* GA 293. Lecture 11.

Examples of affirming with the new-born infant	The more the daily care of the new-born infant is carried out with attention to detail, devotion and love, the more will it in turn feel accepted, valued and loved. This affirmation of the child's being expresses itself through gesture and mime, the sound of the words spoken and each touch of the body. This sounds straightforward, the gesture of affirmation is however difficult to carry through if impatience or irritation surfaces about a screaming and «obstinate» child or if the attentive, comforting and optimistic mood that was intended, falls prey to the daily routine.
with the toddler	Success and failure are part of a toddler's daily life. Its determination and zeal to explore helps it to follow such failure with a redoubling of effort. At this point the child needs affirmation and sometimes comforting too. Adults can be particularly effective in offering comfort and affirmation if they themselves are convinced that the child is capable of overcoming obstacles.
with the kindergarten child	The child completely identifies with its actions and that is why «direct» praise and criticism strongly affects its sense of self and is therefore inappropriate – even when it appears to need it. The child has the right to affirmation even when in the eyes of the educator, it has done something «wrong» or «naughty». A rebuke can and should be given but in such a way that it does not infringe upon the child's sense of self.
What should be considered with regard to affirming?	Praise as a reward for meeting the expectation of the adult offers less effective affirmation to the child than the joy of discovering something beautiful or unexpected in the child's nature. Inflated praise and constant criticism are equally harmful.
What does the child «learn»?	Affirmation and recognition seeds ego power in its being.

Becoming upright

Becoming upright as a gesture	The human being lives between heaven and earth – rooted in the spiritual world he is connected to the earth. Being upright he is free and therefore also responsible. Just as this uprightness is anatomically grounded on the feet, so in the human hand is free creative power expressed. The child attains this upright stature through its own will activity and by imitating sincere and upright people – parents and educators, achieving through its tireless efforts the specifically human capacities of walking, speaking and thinking. These capacities form the basis of the human being's autonomy and social competence.

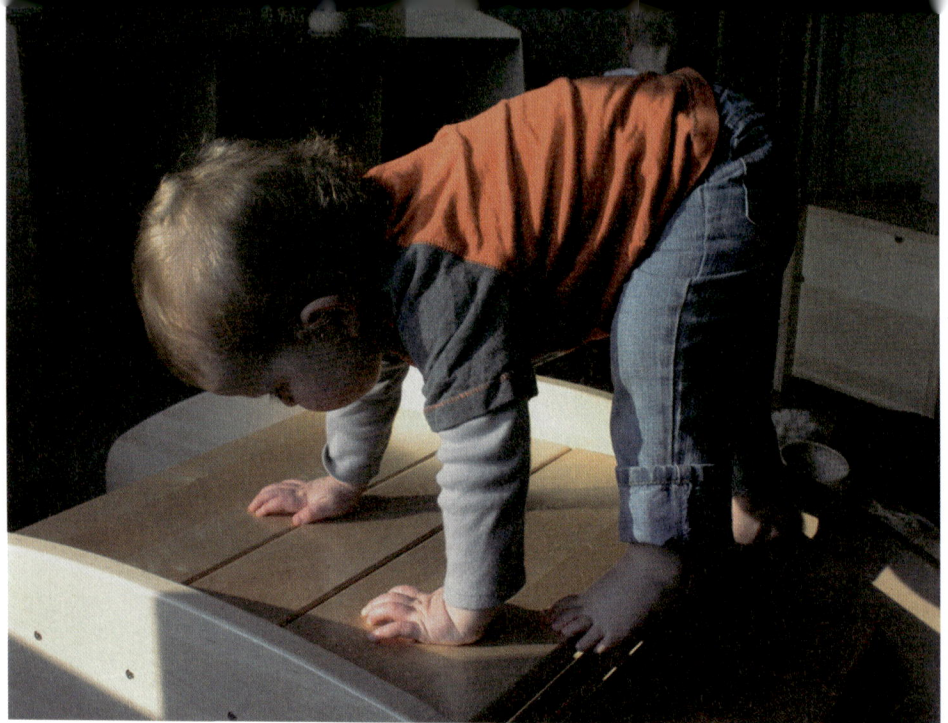

Examples of uprightness with the new-born infant	Even the developing movements of the new-born infant are geared towards walking in the upright position. It is between 12 and 18 months before the child is able to take its first steps. To do so it requires the upright walking example of the person to whom it relates. Out of the lying position it turns on its side, then on the stomach – and lifts its head.
with the toddler	The toddler crawls, sits upright and then scrambles like a bear until it is able to pull itself up on something, holds on while taking its first steps and then walking freely. Becoming upright in this way expresses an autonomy achieved on one's own initiative.
with the kindergarten child	Walking upright is the physiological pre-condition for freeing up the hands and enabling the head to gain an overview of its surroundings. Directed and purposeful actions are now possible. The child becomes skilful with its hands.
What should be considered with regard to uprightness?	The gesture of sincerity assists the process of standing upright. In the case of the new-born infant and toddler physical uprightness is not yet in place. This gesture is primarily carried by the adults internally. It is from there that the forces of uprightness stream. The child seeks orientation and finds it in the uprightness (sincerity) of the main carer.
What does the child «learn» with regard to uprightness?	Uprightness brings about an awareness of human dignity. Through it the child discovers its own uniqueness and worth. Already in encountering setbacks and winning success during its first efforts to move, the child experiences itself as being human. Uprightness is the foundation for freedom and responsibility.

Petra Kühne
Nutrition for the young child

In the first year of life, the child is an infant. Food starts as liquid and is taken in by sucking. At best, this is breast-milk. The recommendations today are 4–6 months full breastfeeding, that means all meals are covered by breast milk. Is breast-feeding not at all possible or only partially possible or only for a shorter time, then the child also receives liquid nourishment: the bottle. Between the 5th and 7th month, the next phase follows: the child moves on to pulpy food. It takes a step towards «firmness», because the pulpy foods are thickened liquids. In addition, food now no longer consists only of a milk base. The child gets the first foods grown on earth, such as carrots, squash or parsnips. This is an important stage on the path of incarnation, of «coming into the flesh», that is, connecting with the earth. The beginning of the pulpy food period should not only be determined according to the age of the child or a tablet of recommendation, but should be made dependent on the stage of development of the child. The pulps require more from the child: they taste and satiate differently, the digestion is more demanding. The child must be ready to accept this new form of meal. A good time for the pulp-phase is when the children begin to move more, become more mobile, roll, turn or crawl. Then their energy and nutrient requirements increase, the child separates spatially more from the mother and moves more independently. This time is between the 5th and 8th month – before the phase of stranger anxiety. The pulpy food is also clearly visible on the diapers: while sometimes nothing is left from a meal of mother's milk, there is now «ballast». The symbiotic food intake via the mother becomes less and the child becomes more self-sufficient even into the digestive system.

The Nutritional-phases

The third nutritional phase is the transition to the first solid food. It starts mostly with the first foods, such as Zwieback, crackers or rice waffles, which they try to «gum» or chew. This is, so to speak, a first trial of the chewing tools and swallowing. Here also, the differences in the children are clear. Some children want this «challenge» to the will (the work of the lower jaw) only later. They chose to enjoy porridges longer, they are consumed without effort. Other children do not care for the pulp; they would like to have what is consumed at the family table. Differences al-

Age of Child	Nutritional-phase	Kind of Food
0–6 month	liquid	Mother's milk, bottle
from 5. (7.) month	semi-firm	pulpy foods
from 9. month to 1 year	firm	first firm food (Zwieback etc.)
1–2 years		introduction to family diet

ready exist in the second half of the year, which will also be reflected in other areas. Sometimes the parents are confused with such a «fast» child, which does not have much enthusiasm for the usual porridge-style, but the preferences show clearly. The child then already eats other foods and along with it, takes a further development step, that occurs later with the porridge-eating children. Still other children take a long time, into the second year, struggling with swallowing problems with small chunks of crackers, pieces of bread and the like. They are only later ready for another diet and often enjoy their porridge long and intensively.

Milk nourishment
Breast milk is completely adapted to the needs of the human child. Every animal food is composed differently. It was not until the 19th century that the various types of milk were analyzed (all mammals produce milk for their offspring). There was a correlation between nutrients and development. The faster an animal child grows, the higher the protein and mineral content in the animal milk. Thus, high protein levels are found in rodents, but also in cats and dogs. Breast milk, on the other hand, has the least amount of protein and minerals. This is a sign of slow physical growth. The child's kidney is also unable to cope with more protein and minerals in the first few months. Recent studies have shown that increased protein content in bottle food promotes the risk of later obesity. However, what breast milk contains in large quantities, unlike almost all types of animal milk, is lactose, (milk-sugar). This easily digestible carbohydrate primarily supplies the brain, that is intensively molded and shaped in the first few years of life. A child never learns more than in the first years of life. The animal milk types are low in lactose except for donkey and horse.

Humans grow slowly physically, take almost two decades to reach the final body size; the mouse offspring can reach it in 6 weeks. This can also be seen from their first food and is a guide for the infant nutrition: Not too much protein and sufficient carbohydrates in good quality. By the way, most of the energy in breast milk is supplied by the fat. Its quality reflects the diet of the mother. If she took in good oils with high proportion of unsaturated fats such as e.g. the omega-3 fatty acid, then they show in the mother's milk. This of course, also applies to the quality of cow's milk. Animals that stand in the pasture or feed on a lot of green food give valuable milk.

Composition of animal- and mother's milk (in %)

	Protein	Fat	Lactose	Minerals
Human	1,2	4,0	7,0	0,2
Horse	2,2	1,5	6,2	0,4
Cow	3,3	3,8	4,7	0,7
Goat	3,7	3,9	4,2	0,8
Sheep	5,3	6,0	4,7	0,9

Source: Souci, Fachmann, Kraut: *The Composition of Foods*. 7. ed. Stuttgart 2008

Today, the quality of livestock farming and feed can even be proven by the nutrients. For this reason Demeter quality (from organic-dynamic cultivation) or organic quality for the food is recommended.

Cow's milk of appropriate quality is a recommended food for children in the second year of life. About 300 ml daily, are enough. This only applies if cow's milk is tolerated – which is the case for 95% of children in Central Europe. It does not have to be just milk, it also includes dairy products such as yoghurt or cream cheese. Quark is recommended only after the 10th month due to the higher protein content. This means that daily a milk porridge / muesli, and one to two slices of bread with cheese or a yoghurt are already sufficient.

The value of the grains

The second staple next to the milk are the grains. They provide the necessary carbohydrates, high-quality vegetable protein and as whole grain it has corresponding vitamins and minerals. It is superior to the potato because of its ingredients and nutritive power and should be used as the satiating component in the porridges. There are various grains; they differ in the ways of cooking, in taste, effect, and tolerability. Spelt, millet, rice, oats and wheat are mainly used in children's foods. They must be prepared accordingly in order to be tolerable for toddlers.

The cereal protein gluten contained in wheat, spelt, rye, barley and some oats can be problematic. More recently it is stated, that when a beginning is made around the sixth to eighth month of life, when there are still some breast milk meals, the risk of an incompatibility is far less. It is therefore not recommended to wait too long to introduce the grain types.

Children's nutrition is easy

In the second year of life, the child gradually gets used to the family meals or the food in the nursery. In these years of life, children have their own nutritional needs that are different from those of adults:
- Children need a regular lifestyle with rhythms.
- Children do not need much variety of foods.
- Children love food of simple composition.

This makes cooking for children easy. Children do not like vegetable mixtures, but just one or two types of vegetables. We should also hold back on spices for a long time, but under no circumstances spices in seed form or kernels (caraway, fennel) should be used in the meals, only finely ground. Government agencies have recently advised that children should get used to many vegetables as early as in the second year of life in order to achieve a diverse diet. This is a challenge for many children, because every vegetable addresses the sense organs differently, and is digested differently. Young children still have plenty of time to get to know the vegetables of the world. This does not have to happen in the first years of life.

Eating should bring joy

What we prepare for the child brings the joys of the immediate physical life, the

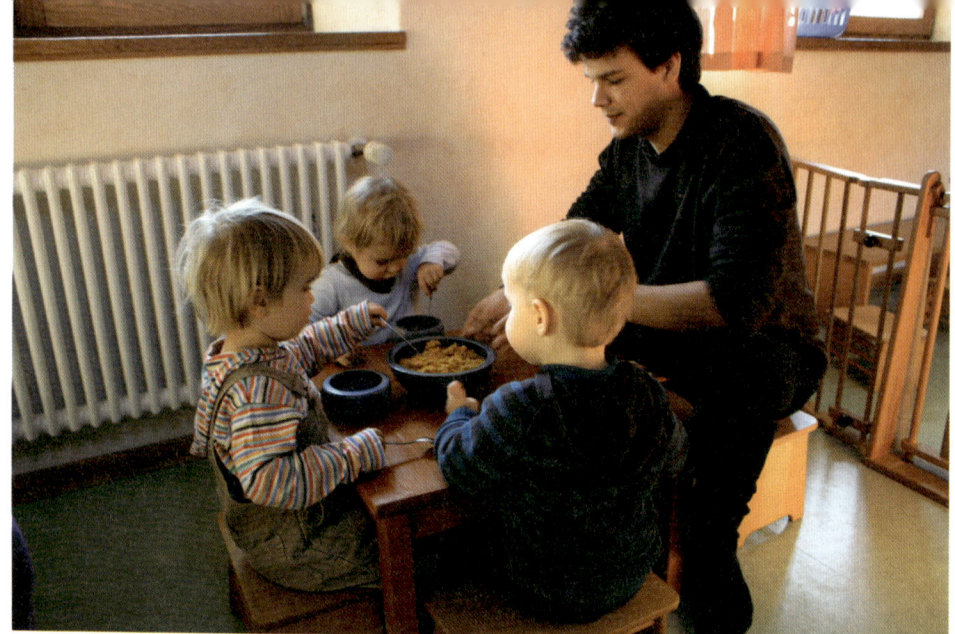

love that flows in from his environment, brings forces to the physical body, that make him capable of learning, that make him, as it were, soft and pliable ...[1]

This statement by Rudolf Steiner's applies, of course, also to food. The meals should be enjoyable and not lead to a power struggle or coercion. Therefore, the fear that children do not eat enough, do not get enough vitamins, etc. when they once refuse to eat vegetables should be avoided. Diet is often seen very abstractly, just intellectually, and the feelings and positive sense-impressions that the child experiences are not perceived enough. Too often scientific nutritional statements have been withdrawn, for example, that children need a lot of spinach or liver to get enough iron. Spinach is not as iron-rich as thought, and liver is rarely recommended for children today because of potential contaminants. Therefore, the observation of children is important without getting too worried about their rejection. Repeated consumption increases the acceptance of the food eaten (Mere Exposure Effect). On the other hand, there is also the specific sensory saturation, if the same food is given too often. Then the children refuse and want something else. However, this takes much longer for young children than for adults. So the food is a learning process in which joy and positive experiences should be in the foreground.

---

1   Rudolf Steiner, *Metamorphoses of the Soul, Paths of Experience*. GA 59, Rudolf Steiner Press, 1983, Lecture from 14.3.1910. Dornach 1972, p. 85.

Brigitte Huisinga
Learning to eat independently in the «Wiegestube»

The topics «Food» and «Nutrition» have become problematic in a time of abundance, with an art of cooking and cooking shows. Allergies and intolerances are increasing. Scientific and popular pedagogical studies and articles confuse parents with contradictory statements.

On the other hand, eating is a sensitive situation for parents and caregivers, because relationship issues are linked with it. Statements such as «cooked with love» or «love goes through the stomach» are well known.

But what does a mother feel when she cooked with love but it is not eaten? What kind of reaction does that cause – disappointment, anger, feelings of inadequacy, …?

When a child does not eat well, parents are worried: they watch carefully to see whether he gains weight, or whether he receives the right nutritional ingredients, they try out what he likes, maybe they run after him with the spoon, begging that he will take a few more spoonfuls. Other children like to eat very much, they want to eat everything they see around as edible immediately – a joy: but will they gain too much wait?

– Julius
Julius, just 1 year old, is to be looked after during the day in the «Wiegestube» (Nursery). The time of parental leave has finished, and both parents are working again. An early and big step for the child, to be passed on from the familiar home situation into unfamiliar hands.

*Will Julius feel comfortable, will the caregivers understand him, will he be able to sleep, and – a frequent and lasting question – will he accept the food?
Later they will have asked: Did he eat and how much?*

For Julius already has preferences, more and more often he is allowed to try the food of his parents, he also wants to eat by himself already, although more lands on the floor than in his mouth, but his parents are happy and respond to his wishes.

Learning to eat in the «Wiegestube»
New children come to the «Wiegestube» with different backgrounds. Most of them spend two years there. During that time they take great developmental steps. They learn to walk securely, to speak and much more; then finally they can also eat independently.

The caregivers are confronted by the expectations of the parents and the particularities of each individual child. During the familiarization period, they get to know the parents and the child and their habits. On the other hand, the parents have the opportunity to experience how and what the children get to eat in the «Wiegestube».

In the search for a way, how a child can learn to eat independently, Emmi Pikler's «Steps to Independent Eating», and the suggestions for a healthy diet by Dr. Kühne, Working Group for Nutrition Research, are a great help. The co-workers of the Wiegestube themselves prepare a tasty meal made from wholesome grains and, if possible, regional produce from the natural food store of the «hof»[1].

– Back to Julius
At home Julius was already allowed to try to eat with his spoon, because the parents want to promote his independence. Even though much is spilled and playing with food is more interesting than putting it in the mouth. The mother quickly slips a spoon full or two in the mouth, so that at least he had something to eat. Both are content in the trusting relationship between mother and child.

In the «Wiegestube», the relationship must be created before the readiness to accept food. Therefore Julius will be fed on the lap of the caregiver during the familiarization time and even after. In the security of being held, the initial narrow ridge of trust becomes ever wider. The caregiver gets to know Julius with his habits:

> How far does he open his mouth?
> Does he want a lot on the
> spoon or only a little?
> Does he eat fast or slow?
> Does he need breaks?

She is talking to him, expressing what she experiences with him or what he expresses through gestures and his physical reactions. For, it is amazing how clearly already the young children can tell us what they want without language: they point with their hands or turn away or reach for the bib when they are done ...

But Julius is not the only child, Lena, Florian and Marie also eat on the laps.

1 Frankfurt «der hof», Alt-Niederursel 51, 60439 Frankfurt, www.der-hof.de.

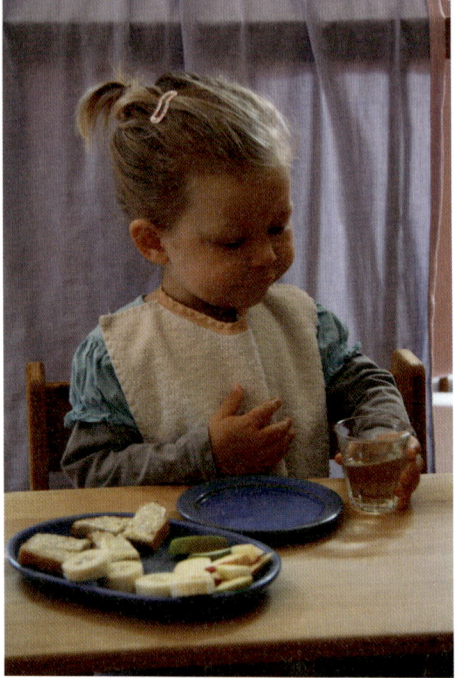

This happens every day at the same time in the same order. After a few days of habituation, all four are sure that they will have their turn, and with a smile, crawl to the caregiver when their turn comes.

«*Eating and drinking should always be a source of joy for the child*» writes Maria Vincze[2] from the Pikler Institute. Joy comes before the what and how much the child eats. In this way, the caregivers in the «Wiegestube» reach the point where all children like to eat well – the best prevention for any eating disorders later in life.

What's next? The child should learn to eat on his/her own, as is customary in our culture in a community.

Eating on the little dining bench
Before Julius can sit at the table with three or four other children, he will learn to eat with a spoon on the little dining-benches and not only that: he learns to stay seated, and not to play with the food but to eat his

2 Maria Vincze, *Schritte zum selbständigen Essen*. Pikler Gesellschaft Berlin 1992, p. 7. (Steps to eating independently)

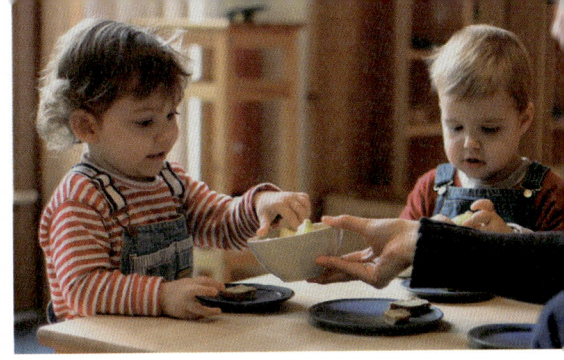

fill. The caregiver helps him mindfully with a second spoon, paying attention to his reactions. Julius climbs all by himself into the dining-bench.

Eating together at the table

For the common meal with several other children at a table new steps of learning are necessary. Julius will have to put up with other children sitting next to him, and to learn that only his own plate is meant for him, and that his spoon should not end up on the neighbor's plate – and he has to «share» the caregiver with the other children. He will experience how nice it is to eat together and have a conversation with the others.

However, the table conversations can only happen when the child does not have to focus anymore on how to handle the spoon. They can also only happen when

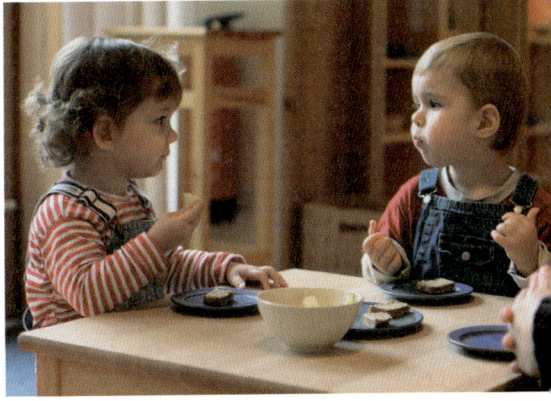

the caregiver does not constantly have to assist but is able to accompany them joyfully and participate in their conversations.

In this way already many philosophical questions are clarified between the children:

«My mommy wears a skirt».
«My mommy is a woman».
«My mommy also wears a skirt».
Theresa: «All mommies are women».

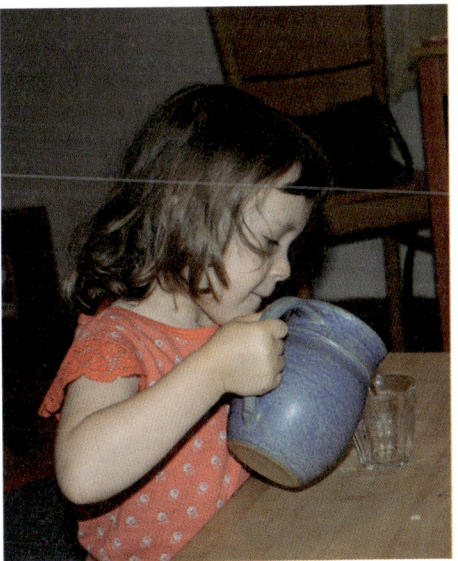

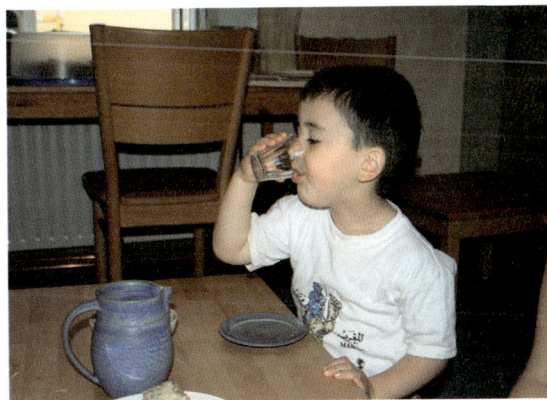

Brigitte Huisinga | Learning to eat independently in the «Wiegestube»

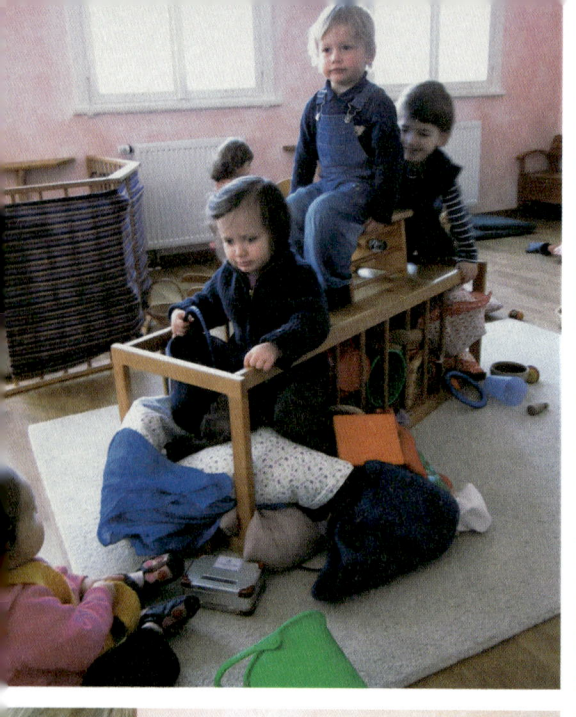
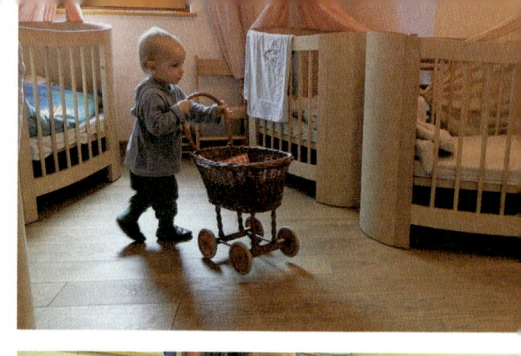
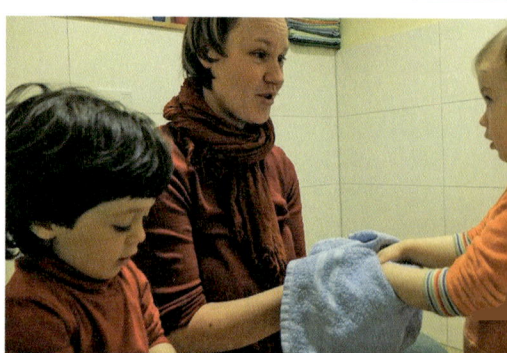
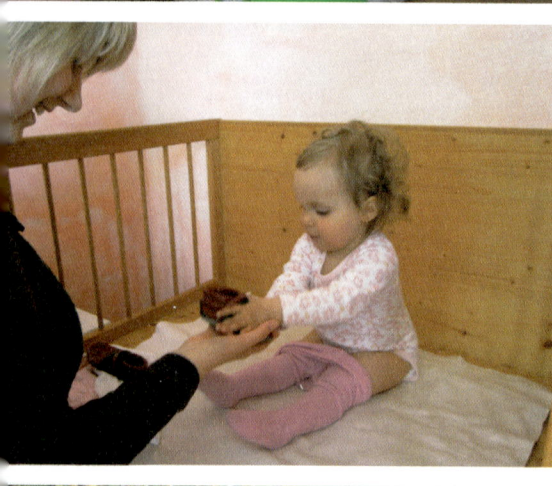
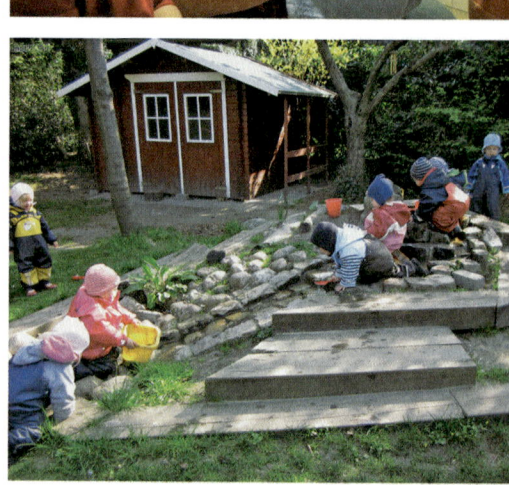
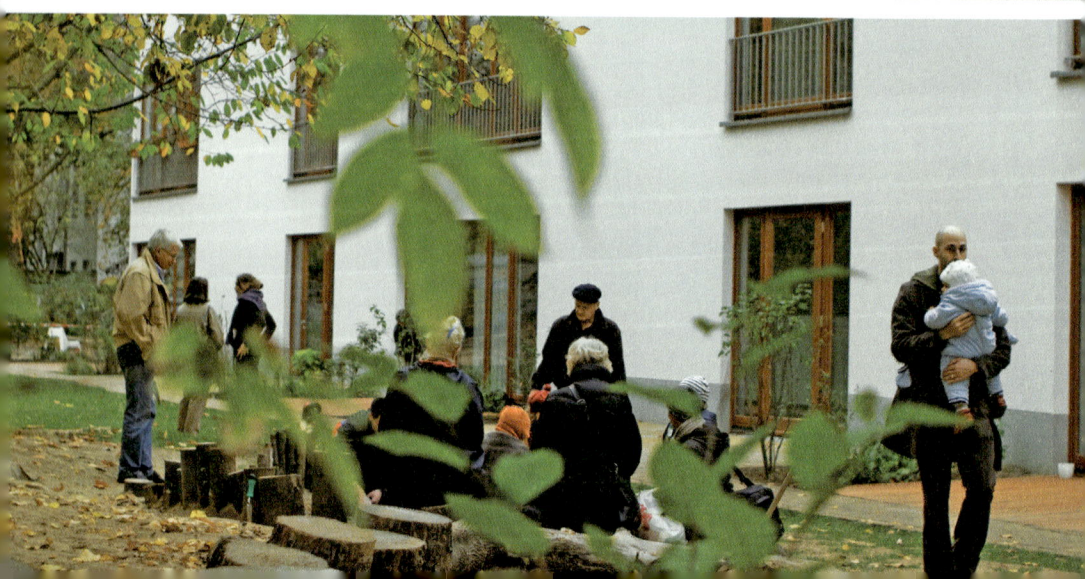

Elisabeth Wutte
Speech development and Speech promotion

The cry is the first sound of the infant. Whether it is due to hunger, discomfort or pleasure is usually recognized only by parents. The cry is the first vocal relationship with the surrounding humans. Crying strengthens the respiratory organs. Only later the smile is added.

In the second year of life, there are blowing games, such as blowing out candles, keeping windmills in motion, table football with cotton balls, but above all singing and rhythmic speech.

In his book on the sense of speech[1], Peter Lutzker points out that the sense of balance acts as an ordering force for all stimulus sensations and thus contributes to the development of the understanding of words and sentences.

For children, the spoken word forms a unity with the lip movements that they see in the speaker. Therefore, many blind children have delayed speech development. Studies show that infants react with discomfort and confusion when in a poorly-synchronized movie the lips and the rest of the body are delayed even only a fraction of seconds to the speech.[2]

Children already hear in the womb. The first lull phase is based on tactile stimuli of the tongue and lips. When the children's «joy of speaking» diminishes after the seventh month of life, the cause may be damage to their hearing. Because, starting with the seventh month of life, the child begins to speak on the basis of hearing. The hearing development itself is completed at about twelve months.

Language and movement

Rudolf Steiner points out the connection between speech and movement. Speech requires the ability to control the movements of the lips and tongue purposefully and willingly. The child acquires the necessary fine motor skills when he has strengthened his muscles, and his joints have become flexible from kicking, turning, crawling, standing, walking, climbing and jumping. There is a relationship between the mobility of the fingers and the ability to speak. Mariela Kolzowa[3] writes, that on the basis of the finger movements we can ascertain the level of speech development – even if we have not heard a single word from the child. Gestures and hand movements have a greater effect on the emotional environment of speech, on the voice and the sound. Free finger movements and differentiated finger plays promote the articulation and the interpenetration of speaking and thinking. They bring awakeness into speech process, whereby the thumb stimulates more the will, and the index and middle finger more the thinking, and the ring and small finger more the artistic feeling. The acquisition of hand and finger skills further the speech development. It can be practiced daily with button-pulling, pyramid-building, painting, folding, kneading dough etc.

---

[1] Peter Lutzker, *Der Sprachsinn. Sprachwahrnehmung als Sinnesvorgang*. Stuttgart 1996. (Sense of word, perceiving speech as a sensory process)
[2] Ibid.
[3] Mariela Kolzowa, *Untersuchungen zur Sprachentwicklung*, Zeitschrift «Der Kinderarzt», 1975/6. (research into the development of speech, Journal: Der Kinderarzt)

Unconscious dancing of speech

Modern kinesics discovered more connections between language and movement: every speaking is accompanied by muscle movements that are so subtle and quick that we do not consciously perceive them. They are so diverse and so intertwined that one can say that our unconscious movement being dances with every word. This is not only the case when speaking – the same process takes place when listening. Speakers and listeners move in a common rhythmic motion stream with only minimal time delay (about 0.4 seconds). Rudolf Steiner has already pointed out – that not only the larynx of both makes the same movements but both movement performers dance the same dance at the same time. This process is the more harmonious, the more the speaker and the listener are in a state of relaxed attention, that is, their general motor activity is in a living balance of activity and rest, tension and relaxation. Since the newborn is already dancing with the word of the person speaking to him, and the so-called imitation is actually a doing together, we encourage the development of the language of the infant and young child, when we are awake and relaxed when we speak to him.

Thus, the speaking human is formed by the muscular mobility of the whole body, and that from birth on, perhaps already in the womb. Some researchers come to the conclusion that the crucial basis for language development is created in the first six months. At the latest after one year, this process is completed, that is, when the child is just starting to speak the first words himself.

In summary, it can be said that language development is proceeding harmoniously when the acquisition of all above mentioned abilities goes hand in hand with movement, that is, sensorimotor integration takes place, which can be linked to thinking. This integration must have taken place by a certain time. For, at the end of the first seven years of life, the sensory apparatus has come to maturity and the brain has reached its final size. Peter Lutzker believes that the intensive language learning phase has now come to a close.

Meeting the language approach of the child

The adult has a manner of speech that is different from the toddler. Our everyday language is rational, informative, communicative. The toddler, on the other hand, discovers sounds, repeats them joyfully, invents words, tells stories in the succession of words. He is touched by voices and responds to them. Our every day speaking in contrast to the child, consists up to 80% of short declarative sentences and commands, like: «Stop that!» «Stay in the chair!» This discrepancy must be overcome.

Some suggestions:
- Listening and letting them speak is an essential prerequisite for children to develop their language skills.
- When we adults start accepting our children's talk and encourage them, even when they speak incorrectly, they gradu-

ally gain confidence in speaking. So do not correct, but annunciate properly. For example: Miti hurt – Oh, did miezi (the cat) hurt you?

- Prepare actions verbally. Language speaks to humans as human beings. Through the spoken word the dignity of the other can be recognized. Emmi Pikler[4] pointed out, that even children with multiple disabilities became able to communicate when they were verbally prepared for the actions performed while caring for them. The important thing is that word and action are closely connected or parallel so that the word does not become abstract. In this way, the spoken word can become a gate for the listener to perceive the thoughts and the personality of the speaker. The listener can then accept more easily the necessities that need to be cared for.
- Our understanding of speech is much greater than our ability to speak, that is, the child understands much more than he can speak. In addition, our upper senses are interwoven with each other, so that while perceiving speech a personal encounter takes place. In speaking, one feels: «*one's own ego in the other's*». «*If he then hears the sound of the other ego, then his own ego lives in this sound and with it in the other's ego*».[5]

- As soon as we can name a feeling, we are no longer helplessly at the mercy of it, but can begin to look at it from the outside. This distancing and describing is a first step in the formation of the consciousness soul, which can already be gently initiated with the small child. Mother says for instance: yes, it annoys you that you cannot pull the shirt over your head. Or: You just hit yourself on the table. That hurts.
- A suggestion to cultivate truthfulness in speaking is given by Rudolf Steiner in the exercise «The right word». In the exercises for the days of the week (Monday). It says:
- «*Only what has sense and meaning should come from our lips … Never speak without a reason! Be gladly silent. Try not to say too much nor too little*».[6]
- When the educator cares about using the right word, it will also be easier for her, to find the right and true word with the child.
- In contrast to the everyday language, children's rhymes and children's poems, have rhyme, rhythm and word creations; they are much closer to the child's speech than our everyday language. The rhyme gives a strong footing to speech with its repetitions of the similar; the rhythm brings a living flow to language, and word creations stimulate close observation and reflection. When speech molds itself into an artistic form, it grows beyond the mere informative.

---

[4] Emmi Pikler, *Friedliche Babys – zufriedene Mütter*. Freiburg 1999, 9. ed. (Peaceful Babies – Contented Mothers)

[5] Rudolf Steiner, *Anthroposophy – A Fragment*. GA 45, Chp. Concerning hearing and speaking. Dornach 1951, p. 160 f.

[6] Rudolf Steiner, *Meditations for the Time of Day and Seasons of the Year*. GA 267. Rudolf Steiner Press, 2018.

As poetry, it receives extra power, something rounded and uplifting. Example: You have done well. Or: Exactly, exactly, you are so smart!

Children's rhymes and Children's verses (in German)

For centuries there have been children's rhymes and children's verses for all life situations:

- – Kribbelmaren und Kosesprüche: «Kommt der Bär, der tappt so schwer …» Berühren einzelner Körperteile
- Handmaren: «Da hast 'nen Taler …» Berühren der Handinnenfläche
- Trösterchen: «Heile, heile Segen …»
- Kniereiter: «Hoppe, hoppe Reiter …»
- Fingerspiele: «Das ist der Vater lieb und gut …»
- Auszählverse, Ringelspiele, Rätsel, Nonsens: «Ene, mene miste …»; «Ri ra rutsch, wir fahren mit der Kutsch …»
- Alltagssprüche, z.B. zum Kochen, Waschen, Leise-Werden: «Backe, backe Kuchen …»
- Verwandte, Bekannte, Gesellschaftspolitisches: «Mutter, schaff Butter, Vater, schaff Taler, dass die Mutter die Butter kann zahlen …»;
- Belastendes, Sehnsüchte, Spott: «Lott is dot, Lott is dot, Jule liegt im Sterben, dat is got, dat is got, kriegn mer wat zu erben.»

The children's verses are time-based and not as objective as the fairy tale. That is why we have to write new children's sayings related to our lives.

An example of this is a blessing that came about through a separation situation:

The shirt too short
The wings trimmed
Through the house the wind
God bless you, child.

In the epilogue of *Allerleirauh* (Grimm's: *All kinds of Fur*), Hans Magnus Enzensberger writes that the nursery rhyme belongs to the poetic subsistence minimum of a person and a folk, and through it often lights up the ubiquity of poetry. Perhaps that is why the nursery rhyme has such a strong, incorruptible life. May this continue into the future!

Language development

Since the language development is very individual, the following age specifications are only to be taken as average values; they can shift up to half a year.

Age	Linguistic expression and Language comprehension
1st year of life	Crying as expression of different needs. Cooing in different pitches. (i.e. expression of well-being). Lulling (tactile stimulus). Reactions to tones and noises. Language comprehension not yet verifiable.

3–6 months	Laughing, screeching, cooing. First lulling phase: First sounds: gr..gr, ech...ech. These are international, i.e. you find similar sounds with children of all nations. Through this foreign languages can be learned later on. They startle from sudden noise, turn head to speech- or source of noise. Language comprehension not yet verifiable.
6–9 months	Syllables and syllable doubling (dada, baba). Tries out vocal registers. Listens to his own voice, word-comprehension begins, in context with tone, facial expressions and gestures.
9–12 months	Speaks at least one word, perhaps already 10 words. Parrots words, syllables without context of meaning. Responds to his own name, follows small requests, such as: give it to me. The child learns by praise and encouragement to distinguish whether a word makes sense or is a sound-picture.
2nd year of life	The second year of life is characterized by the development of the spoken word. It is the speech and language year of the child.
12–18 months	One word sentences. The child asks or negates, wishes something with one word with a different speech melody. «Mommy» means a lot, like: «Mommy come; I'm thirsty; I want to sleep». Focus on sound-formation. The child hears the individual sound and reads it from the lips. Therefore, the first conscious sounds are lip sounds: m, b, p. These are linked to vocabulary. The child enjoys rhymes and imitates animal sounds. Responds to requests from a small distance (about one meter).
18–24 months	Two word sentences. Daddy away. Mi (l) ch d (r) ingen. (drink milk) In addition to nouns, action words and adjectives are also used (63% nouns, 23% verbs, 14% adjectives), according to Karl König, *The first three years*[7]). Sentences are unformed. Words stand side by side: Lisa fall (s) tul. First questioning age. Focus on sound formation. Shaping of the dental lip sounds w and f and the tooth sounds d, t. Naming phase. The things are named. The word becomes name. At 24 months, the child knows about 250 words. The passive vocabulary is far ahead of the active vocabulary. Responds when he hears his name, from 4 to 6 meters away.

---

[7] Karl König, *The First Three Years of the Child – Walking, Speaking, Thinking*. Second revised edition. Floris Books, 2004.

3rd year of life	Three word sentences. Subject, predicate, objects are used with the first usage of the ego-form, mostly still in the infinitive. First sub-clauses. Time of W- questions begins. Sound formation. Articulately, most sounds are mastered, but not all sound connections, e.g. kn, bl, gr. Also the sibilants (ch, sch, s) do not need to be mastered yet. Explosion of vocabulary. Word creations that are stimulated by thinking-along, e.g. car beep beep (airplane). Example of speech: There is (t) ne F (r) au, (there is a woman) who looks out of the window. Why? Everyday language is understood except for finer gradations (for example, large-larger), foreign words and unknown objects.
4th year of life	Formation of complex sentences with subordinate clauses. Only difficult sentence constructions are faulty. The child begins to tell, who, what, where, when, and why, and uses plural and past. Control of all sounds except occasionally for sibilants and more difficult consonant compounds, such as street (steet) or plum (German: pflaume -plaume).
5th year of life	Vocabulary is growing; pronouns and colors are used. The child can form all sounds without mistakes. Forms sentences of 5 words, masters the tenses and tells what he has done during the day. He asks for the meaning of words that he does not know. The mother tongue is mastered with the feeling. If, at the end of the age of five, there is still a speech problem concerning the forming of sound-, of word- or sentence formation, a physician or speech therapist should be consulted.

Brigitte Huisinga
Speech development through connection

Learning to speak is not an act of training, but a natural process in a child's development which means more than just learning to speak.

Even newborns are attentive when we speak to them. It is as if they were drinking in the language. Being addressed conveys to them: «I take you seriously, I speak to you. I am with you». To this and to eye contact, they react from the beginning.

Even if an infant does not yet understand the words, it is important to speak to him normally. By doing so, I show what image I have of the child, that I regard him as a full-fledged human being and as a worthy partner.

Speaking during care-taking

When care-taking, diapering, dressing, feeding, it is important to speak to the child to transmit mindfulness and respect. Carefully «handling» him, while he himself remains passive, but not telling him what is happening, is not respectful. We should therefore tell him before the care-taking activities, what will happen with him/her, what we will be doing, and what we expect of her/him.

The child needs time to react, and s/he reacts differently according to age and ability: with a slight movement, a little gesture, with a smile or with sounds. Then we can adjust ourselves, and in this way an exchange happens. This «conversation» develops into a very personal relationship.

The actual availability and joy of the adult, her smile, the tender and joyful reciprocal exchange and the times of

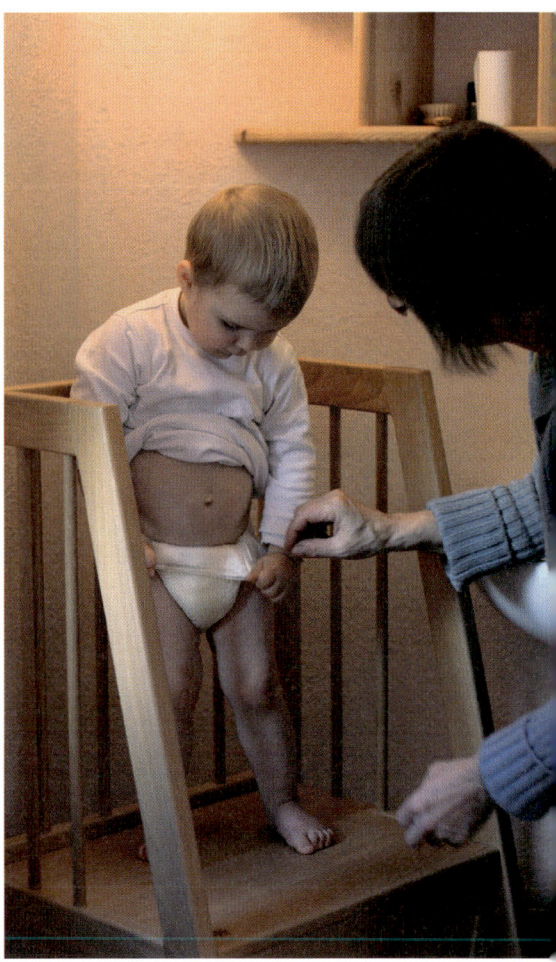

waiting, create an atmosphere in which the child feels that it is worthwhile being loved. That forms the basis of his/her self-esteem.[1]

---

1 Ute Strub, Anna Tardos (ed.), *Im Dialog mit dem Säugling und Kleinkind*. Pikler Gesellschaft Berlin 2006, p. 28. (In conversation with infants and young children)

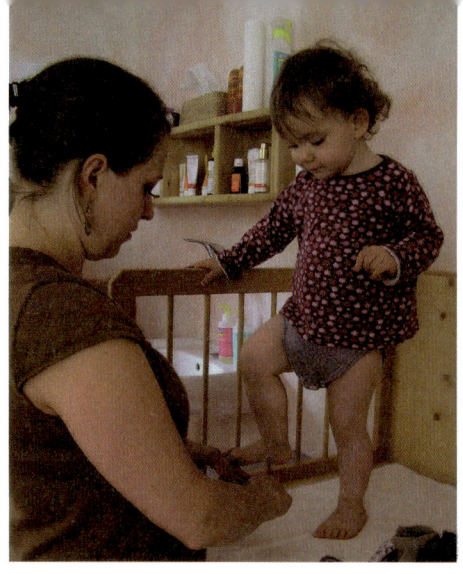

Talking to the toddler

The toddler chats, s/he speaks to us. There is a big difference in the way the sound is expressed, whether the child plays and at the same time makes sounds, i.e. long sequences of da, da.., or whether s/he is on the diaper table in a conversation with the caregiver. Here, the sounds are rather short, like he is waiting for an answer, so to speak.

Speaking with the child when we take care of him/her, is not only important for the child's relationship and self-esteem, but is crucial to the language development. It is not enough for language acquisition when the child only hears what is spoken all around him, he must experience that he is being addressed.

The child learns to speak from the adult, therefore it is especially important how we speak with him – meaning not purposefully slow or with exaggerated exactness: We should speak clearly, grammatically correct, in a simple way, with a calm flow, friendly, no baby talk, always trusting that the child will understand.

When the child is a bit older and can already speak some words, he begins to tell us something. He names his body parts, talks about his clothing, about what he sees, and what he has experienced. Everything depends on our sensitivity, on our effort to understand what he would like to tell us. Here follows a conversation with Marie:

«You are wearing two different socks».
«Gone».
«You couldn't find the second sock this morning»?
«Martin search».
«Martin searched for the sock, but could not find it, so he just put another one on you».
«Yes!»

Marie is radiant. She feels that she has been understood.

In an engaging relationship with the child, the dialogue always becomes richer. This is how the child learns to speak with pleasure!

Marie-Luise Compani
Leaving the Crèche

Transitions accompany us humans for a lifetime. Taking leave, separating, embracing new experiences, and new relationships are all part of the human biography. Transitions always represent a break with what is familiar, well-known and dear. The security of the old is given up for something new and unknown. Thus, treading «new territory» is always a sensitive phase.

Many of today's children experience their childhood as a succession of out of the familiar child – caring forms which means that an essential part of childhood is given into the responsibility of institutions. This starts at infant age with the crèche, later to be followed by the kindergarten, and during school-time, the child spends part of his/her free time in after-care. The transitions from one institution to another are added to the individual, biography-based transitions, like moving and/or separation of parents.

Educators and parents have the task and the responsibility to prepare these transitions for the child carefully and with sensitivity, so that the changing environment and relationships do not have a negative effect on the child's development.[1]

The expansion of early child care in the old Bundesländern (German states) is rapidly increasing. In the founding euphoria it is often overlooked that the change to kindergarten must also be pedagogically accompanied, just like the acclimatization period in the crèche.

Educational Aspects

There are a number of pedagogical aspects that are based on the development and well-being of the child. Above all, the age-related development of the child and not his/her age should be the criterion for switching to kindergarten. The following criteria must be observed:
- degree of independence that has been acquired, such as eating independently
- socio-emotional maturity: How much closeness does the child still need? Can s/he separate himself from the educator?
- speech development
- movement development
- play development.

Newland kindergarten and familiarization

If there is a close, spatial contact between the two facilities, there is often an opportunity during free play in the garden, to casually get to know the caregivers and the children. Then the kindergarten is at least not completely foreign to the child from the point of view of the spatial conditions.

In case of a solitary crèche (infant care facility) without a connection to a kindergarten, the spatial change can be a big step for the child. The new orientation means for the child, different habits, rules, rituals to get used to. The groups in kindergarten are as a rule, twice as large as in the crèches. Children experience a group three times as big as it actually is. A child who

---

[1] See Hans-Joachim Laewen, Beate Andres, Eva Hedervari, *Die ersten Tage – ein Modell zur Eingewöhnung in Krippe und Tagespflege*. Beltz-Verlag 2003; the same: *Ohne Eltern geht es nicht: Die Eingewöhnung von Kindern in Krippen und Tagespflege*. Berlin 2006. (the first days – a model for acclimatizing to the play group and day care)

enters into a group of twenty children, experiences this as a gathering of 60 people. There is a much higher noise level that can be experiences as turmoil. The child has to orient himself anew for, the space is equipped with new and different play materials. The daily routine is adjusted in its timing and content to the needs of the older children. The child, new to kindergarten, is therefore dependent on the help and support of a person, who can give him security, protection and company for the transition time.

From the afore mentioned points we can see, that also in kindergarten a familiarization time is needed, so that the child can form a relationship to the responsible educators. In this process, parents are the vital partners and should play a part in it from the beginning. Similar to the crèche, the kindergarten also needs a familiarization concept and attending conversations. From studies it is known that children are more susceptible to sickness when the familiarization is insufficiently accompanied by the parents.

In a concluding conversation at the end of the familiarization period, parents and educators together should reflect on the beginning time in the kindergarten. In this way, both sides are assured that the child has now fully arrived, feels well and protected.

Practical indications to structure the farewell

Every separation is at the same time a good bye. This is also the case for the young child, when he changes to kindergarten. A short good bye ritual that emphasizes this transition which is the end of the time in infant care, is helpful for the child and his parents, in order to take this step actively. This can find expression in a small gift for the child and a card for the parents. The packing of the personal things, like house shoes, additional clothing, the cuddle bear that accompanied the child at nap-time, all this makes the transition clearer and more tangible.

In some crèches, that are directly attached to a kindergarten, children may visit the future kindergarten group by the hour, accompanied by an educator. In this way, the child can become familiar step by step with the kindergarten group. However, this accompaniment should not replace the familiarization period with the parents in the kindergarten; however, this can be shortened in this way. Since the familiarization time of each child is very individual, this process requires transparency and trust in working together with colleagues.

– Exchange with parents

The transition to kindergarten must be carried out in partnership with all concerned. The exchange between educators and parents about the development of the child must take place *before* that. A retrospective conclusion about the time spent in the crèche offers a possibility to look once again intensively at the development of the child, but also to ease the worries of the parents about the transition to kindergarten.

Of course, there will also be an admission conversation with the educators of the kindergarten. Here the familiarization time with the parents will be considered, and it will be pointed out that the children changing from the crèche will also need a familiarization time.

– Working together with colleagues

The collaboration between educating colleagues in pedagogical questions builds the foundation for the mutual appreciation of the different areas of responsibility. These areas of responsibility are mirrored in the different concepts of crèche and kindergarten.

In the kindergarten the child gradually develops a sense of community – s/he breaks away from his self-concern and becomes sociable. He can now exist in a larger group of children alone, without the need for immediate adult attention. In addition to free play, various activities are of increasing importance.

– Transitioning to the kindergarten

Moving on to the kindergarten takes place as a rule, on the third birthday of the child. This has an impact on the structure of the institution: it brings with it a constant coming and going within the group, for available places must be filled quickly for financial reasons.

It is therefore advisable, to clarify the duration of the subsidization of the place in the crèche by the commune, before the opening of the crèche/nursery and then to adjust the conception of the nursery to it. In most cases, there will be a range of about three months for the transition. Not all three-year olds have to change into the kindergarten immediately. One or the other will have the possibility, if necessary for various reasons to catch up with the maturation process within the smaller situation of the crèche.

Another possibility would be, to carry out the transitioning at the end of the kindergarten year, and a second agreed upon transition time – e.g. after Christmas or Easter, in order to avoid a constant fluctuation in the group.

As soon as the young children's groups are affiliated with a kindergarten, they influence the admittance-structure of the kindergarten. As a rule, new children are admitted after the summer holidays. In order that the children from the crèche can change in the course of the year, there must be places available otherwise the kindergarten group will be over the limit. There needs to be a timely and workable agreement between crèche and kindergarten, so that all nursery/crèche children can be admitted into the kindergarten.

Claudia Grah-Wittich
Working together with parents

The younger the child, the more is s/he still directly connected with the thinking and the life of his immediate environment, especially with his closest caregivers – his parents. Today, there are many additional care options and care-facilities. Since 1. August 2013, and with expenditures into the billions, the legal entitlement to a childcare place for children ages 1 – 3, has now grown to almost full coverage (in Germany) for day care options for the youngest, who sometimes are only a few months old. They are with day-mothers, in crèches, cradle-or crawling-places and whatever names they have. This is in addition to the existing Kindergartens and Kinder-day-care-places.

As a result, parental work gains a new status in the institution, as mothers and fathers have given over the immediate responsibility for their child and his development for many hours each day – and yet they still remain absolutely responsible for his/her well-being.

> *How can parents and institutions work together optimally in the child's best interests?*
> *How is the human interaction formed between the parents as the primary caregivers of the children and the professionally trained educators?*

The pre-school years, and especially the first three years, have a unique significance for the entire life of the child and his possibilities, for better or worse. Anthroposophic study of the human being and the latest scientific findings are fully consistent on this point. Decisive for the future development of an independent personality is the way *how* walking, speaking and thinking were learned, and how the whole body building and shaping was able to unfold.

Children are exposed to their environment

As an adult, one notices quickly the permeability and malleability of children, not only by our actions, but above all through our feeling and thinking. Children live completely in the perception of their environment. Here the example of a three-year-old: in the evening, after his son spend a day in the crèche, the father asks, and the mother talks about the situation she experienced with the delivery and pick-up. The three-year old boy, seemingly not participating in the conversation, but deeply involved in playing with his truck, speaks up and says, as if on the side: «Mommy does not like Mrs. XY». Children before the third year of life – before they can separate themselves off from the world through their own I – have an immediate access to the world, to the environment. Even if many do not constantly reflect this, but keep it more inside, we should, nevertheless, bring to our consciousness as parents/adults what our connection to the surrounding world is. Our relationship to the world imprints itself strongly on the child and will be reflected in his later relationship to his social environment, influencing his social integrity. How this process is established and supported in the parental home and facility and their collaboration is of great importance.

Self-education and self-reflection will become more and more important in the future as the tools for parents as well as for the pedagogical occupations in early childhood. These abilities will find their way into the training as necessary foundation for a qualified educator. The developing human being is at the center of Waldorf education; to work with him in a conscious and developmentally appropriate way is the challenge and task of parents and educators.

A paradigm change is noticeable: In addition to educational questions and to questions concerning the development of the child, adults will, as the primary environment of the child, need to concern themselves with questions of self development and guide their attention more strongly towards themselves: This pausing and becoming aware of one's own responsibility, is like a spark, a moment of freedom to change one's own conduct. The ego is required to become an inner observer and «master in the house» in the sense of a role model. If I deal in a mindful and respectful way with my own feelings, I will develop interest in the situation and the differentness of the other.

The knowledge of these relationships is the inner basis for parent work and parent participation in facilities based on Waldorf education and anthroposophy.

The relationship between parents and institution

The changed living conditions and the increasing individuation of parents brings about that now between 50 to 60% of three-year-olds, and over 90% of the children older than three-years (in Germany) are looked after institutionally, of these, around one third full time. Still, the parents remain the most important care-takers for the child, even if s/he spends the day mostly in an infant care facility or kindergarten. The child perceives subliminally and very well what the relationship of mother or father is towards the facility, and how they experience the atmosphere – and s/he orients himself accordingly.

The relationship between home and institution is well-defined in the legal framework for this care, the «Children- and Youth Welfare Act»: «*The range of services provided by the institutions should be oriented pedagogically and organizationally to the needs of children and families.*»[1]

Based on the psychologist Michael Lukas Moeller, the following professional basic maxims could be formulated for institutions in the field of child care:

I cannot change the parents home or parent «... *If it were possible, I should not even do it; because it would be an attack, a violation of his human rights. I can change myself, my views. If I'm lucky, the relationship will then change as well*».[2]

For caretakers in relation to the parental work this means:
- constantly reflect on your own role behavior
- to feel and communicate soul perceptions and sensations well

---

1 See § 22, 2 KJHG.
2 Michael Lukas Moeller, *Die Wahrheit beginnt zu zweit*. Reinbek bei Hamburg 1995. (Truth begins together)

- to stay with yourself, do not impose your own ideas on others.

If the leaders and caregivers in an institution practice of these qualities, it also will be easier for parents, to remain at ease in their role as parents and to take responsibility for themselves. They will express their own perceptions and feelings concerning their child's situation in the institution appropriately, conscious of the shared responsibility for the well-being of the child.

Attachment and caregiver in a facility

Since the 1970s, we know from numerous studies of attachment research – recently confirmed by insights from neurology and brain research – that the starting point for the development of the child and his independent conquest of the world, is the secure basis of at least one parent.[3] This basis results from the emotional bond. As research and practice show, with the appropriate design and familiarization, adding another caregiver in an institution is entirely possible and, in many situations, necessary and even beneficial to the child.

Nevertheless, the parents always remain the parents and caregivers in the facility the mindful substitutes. A child – and especially a small child – must always be seen in the context with their parents and the respective caretaker: The caretakers implement this concretely by inwardly placing the parents next to them when they take care of the child. This is a fundamental and unconditional requirement for quality of care.

The inner attitude is decisive

When dealing with children the perception of the more delicate signals that often leave a lasting effect, must be trained. Caregivers need to learn the mindful handling of human encounters. It is about the inner attitude that every human encounter is a unique experience, and as caregiver one needs to meet it in a unique way as well. Every encounter is a first encounter! If we do not succeed in developing this attitude, the other person does not feel understood.

In the cooperation between parents and caregivers, it is necessary to work continuously on this inner attitude.

In order to achieve a successful parental participation, all participants need qualities to increase their emotional awareness:

1. Presence

It is necessary to be present if human encounters are to happen. When we meet, each participant notices immediately if the other person is really interested. If fears, insecurities and defensiveness make us avoid direct contact with the other person – then I am with my fears and not with the other person. Openness requires courage: I give up my protection and get involved in the encounter immediately.

2. Authenticity

My counterpart immediately notices if my statements and my actions are in line with my feelings and thoughts. A seemingly

---

[3] See Karl Gebauer, Gerald Hüther, *Kinder brauchen Wurzeln*. 5. ed. Düsseldorf/Zürich 2005. (Children need to have roots, new perspectives for a successful development)

factual concern may not be properly taken in and understood, even if it is presented in a very friendly manner, if I feel irritated, am angry, or feel grief in me. Either I succeed to be the master over my feelings or I speak about my feelings, my concerns and my unfulfilled needs. Only in this way can a space be created for mutual understanding.

3. Respecting the other

In a cooperative partnership mistakes are made and it is alright to make mistakes. It is crucial to stay in dialogue. Everyone wants to be valued in their work and as a personality, irrespective of mistakes or of belonging to another culture or religion and irrespective of other norms and other weighted values. This is extremely important for free conduct with one another. Appreciation always refers to the person irrespective of their behavior.

4. Empathetic communication

Authenticity and the ability to be totally centered and present, are the prerequisites for being empathetic. When I am centered in myself, I can respond to others and show sympathy and interest – then I am also appreciative. Out of this develops naturally the empathetic communication, the ability to perceive attentively the needs and statements of the other, without bringing our own emotional aspects and images into it.

These qualities will change every contact between parents and educators positively – every relationship as such.

Ria Blom
When Babies often cry

Most parents sense more or less how healing rhythm and predictability is for young children.

But how do you implement that concretely?

Should I give something to drink immediately when s/he wakes up or just before putting him to bed?

Does it matter if the child is put to bed when asleep or when still awake?

Does it make a difference whether the child goes to sleep in his own cradle or in the playpen, or in a baby bouncer?

Parents often see no connection between these questions and rhythm and predictability. For the baby, however, proceeding in the «right» way, makes a difference like day and night.

Difficulties of parents

Each child should be given the necessary time to proceed along their own speed of development. However, many children are already put down to play, although they do not sit up by themselves. Or they are taken by the hand, although they cannot stand up by themselves yet. In this way, we take away from the child the wonderful opportunity to experience what it means to come into the up-right on his/her own accord at the right time.

The consequence of this is that children are increasingly demanding attention and play less and less alone. Before the parents understand what is happening, their child has turned into a princess or a prince who swings the scepter:

The child determines now when and if he wants to sleep or not.

Due to the lack of structure and the insecurity of the parents, the child gets used to less and less sleep: he is increasingly over-stimulated and goes far beyond his limits. For example, an unruly two-year-old foregoes his indispensable noon sleep.

Babies without rhythm increasingly start to whine, cry and sleep less because they are simply over-tired. Newborns sometimes cry much of the day, and some older children are so restless, that we refer to them as «restless children».

Joy, calm and trust should be the basic mood after birth. But often, the whole family is completely confused after three weeks, because the baby won't go to sleep: The overtired child receives much attention, he is lovingly carried around until he falls asleep, and when he finally falls asleep after being carried for a long time and carefully placed in his own bed, (or in that of his parents), he immediately starts crying again.

Where do the many restless children come from?

How can joy and trust be won again when living with a baby?

How can parents regain their sound intuition?

Rhythm and predictability are the remedies that can be supplemented up to the age of six months during sleep by swaddling. In the forties and fifties there were still the «three Rs» (in German) of «calm, regularity und purity» as the mainstay of raising children. We left these qualities behind a long time ago. Young parents are insecure and often «they do not see the trees for all the forest» – they are overwhelmed by an overkill of information. Lack of limits and lack of rules in the daily rhythm are the main causes of the restlessness in children.

Above all, my method is based on the application of the «four Rs»: rest, (predictable and unambiguous) regularity, respect and direction.

Foreseeable regularity

Foreseeable regularity means the events at home or in the infant care facility have the same order or as far as possible:
- drink after waking up
- then cuddle in your arms or lap
- then play alone at a certain, defined place (from 4 weeks on)
- in case of signs of tiredness put to bed awake

After a short while the child knows that waking up means: «Now I am allowed to drink». When lifted up after playing, this means: «Now I am allowed to sleep». This gives the child security. He knows what will happen and what can be expected, and he moves more easily with the flow of the day.

By the way, one should not confuse this accustoming with pampering. You can really spoil a baby only after six months.

Lotte Mare – Parents report:
«The first week after her birth, Lotte Mare sleeps during the day and in the evening mainly on daddy's or mommy's tummy. At night, she sleeps during those first weeks in her own bed and with 8 weeks, she sleeps without interruption.

Then she starts to sleep less during the day; She is more active and would like to follow and experience everything that happens around her. When she is three months old, sometimes she only sleeps for one and a half hours during the whole day. This is far too short for her. She becomes increasingly restless, drinks only very little, goes to sleep briefly and wakes up because she is hungry – a devil's circle!

Going to sleep becomes an ever greater problem – we pace around the whole house with her, sometimes in a sling, or we sit next to her bed, while she sucks on our little finger. Lotte Mare does not want a pacifier, and since we fed her milk with a finger for the first days, she got used to suck on her little finger. Every now and then we turn on the hairdryer because that calms her down.

After our summer holidays, we had enough. Lotte Mare is four months old, mother and father have back problems – walking around is out of the question. We are both too tired, and we are beginning to understand that we taught Lotte Mare unintentionally bad sleep habits. The greatest problem is that she cannot go to sleep».

As these parents of Lotte Mare, many parents find it difficult to put their baby to bed while still awake. They let the child go to sleep on their lap and then carefully put him to bed. Perhaps he sleeps well the first one or two weeks, but then this probably changes. It takes ever longer, till the child goes to sleep on the arm, and the sleep becomes ever shorter. It can take months till the well-intentioned parents become aware that their eager child is too tired. The way back is not easy.

All children need rest, rhythm, warmth, security – and very much sleep.

Swaddling

When parents keep to the new rules of life, of the «four Rs» – quiet, regularity, respect and direction – they discover to their surprise, that their baby needs much more sleep than they thought. Warmer, and yet not too warm clothing, a fastened blanket and consequent regularity during the day work like wonder. When the baby continues with the sleeping problems even when using the «four Rs», swaddling can provide the necessary restraint. This makes it easier for the child to go to sleep. Before going to sleep, he/she is wrapped in two sheets, covering and enveloping him. This limiting promotes the development of the tactile sense and the sense of life. It also supports the warmth organization.

Swaddling should be considered as a temporary measure that can help to bring rest to the overly tired child. It should be a tool to introduce and establish a fixed rhythm.

When should you not swaddle?
- by hip dysplasia
- during a fever
- in the first 24 hours after vaccination
- when the baby is 6 months old
- The wrapped child tries to turn on the stomach, although cloths and bed are accurately wrapped and arranged.

To set physical limits and boundaries lovingly belongs together and complements each other in education.

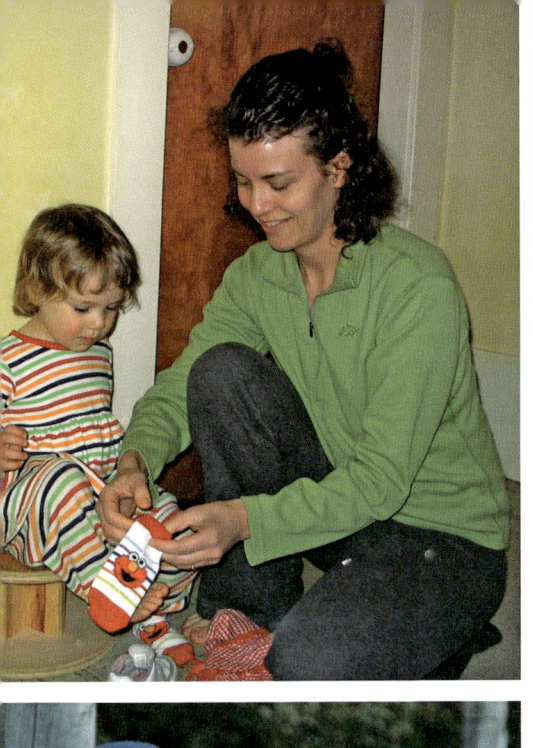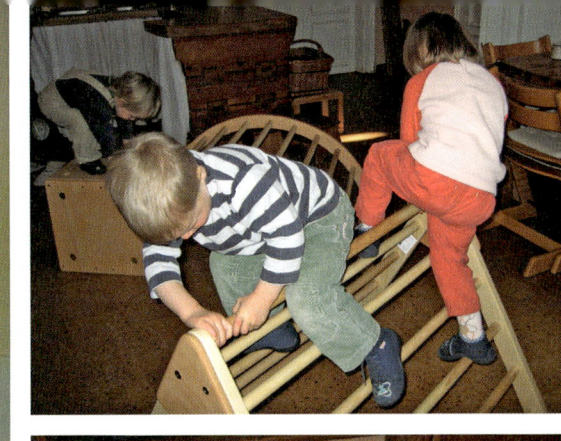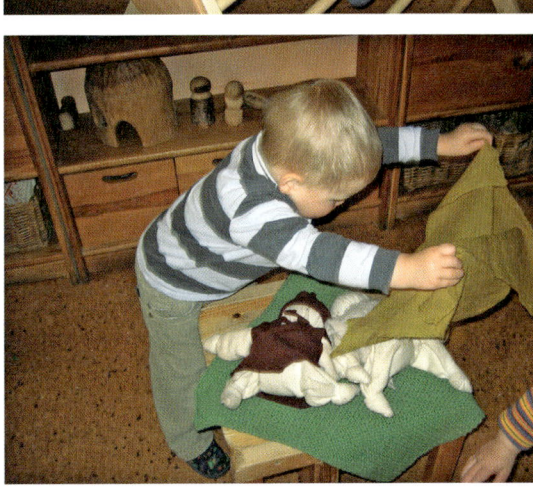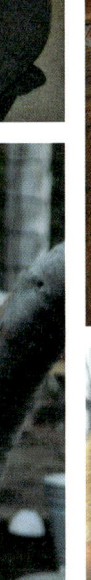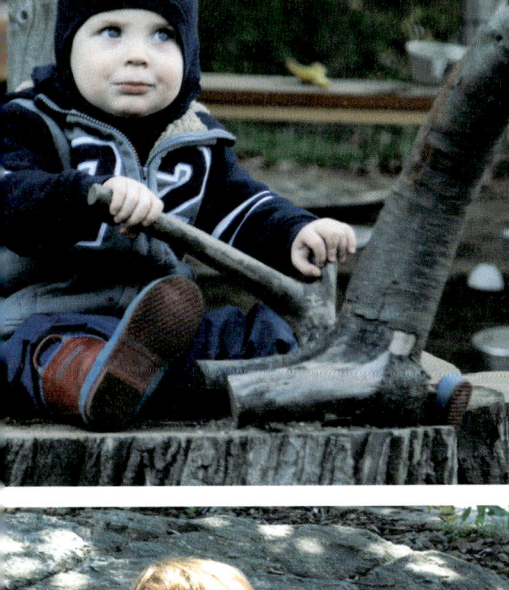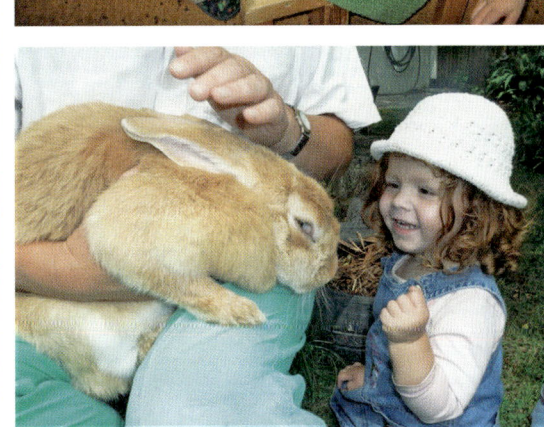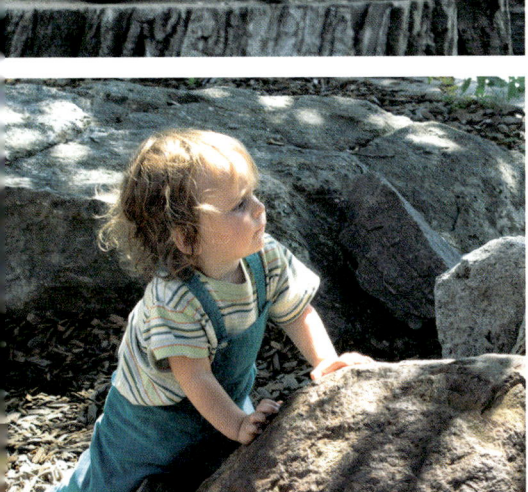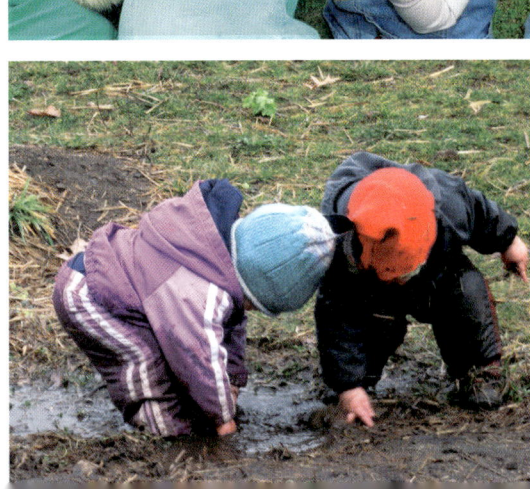

Madeleen Winkler
Mistreatment and neglect

In Holland 15% of women and 2% of men admit that they had «bad» experiences (abuse) before their 16th year of life. 30 to 60% of men and women who seek psychotherapeutic and psychiatric help suffered some form of abuse. 10% of children, one out of 10 children, go through experiences of abuse, mistreatment and/or neglect. 3% of old people are mistreated or abused. Even anthroposophic establishments (schools, kindergartens, practices) are not exempted. In order to recognize abuse, we must know the symptoms.

Forms of mistreatment

- *Physical mistreatment:* The child is beaten or tormented
- *Sexual mistreatment:* Incest, sexual assaults
- *Physical neglect:* The child is malnourished, not dressed according to the season, not washed, not cared for, does not get love nor affection and much more.
- *Soul mistreatment:* The child is scolded. What today is permitted, will tomorrow be forbidden. There are high expectations that the child cannot fulfill yet. The father for example, wanted to study the piano, but was not allowed to do so. Now the child shall study piano, however, she does not like it, but has to practice for hours. It is precisely this psychological mistreatment that we find in all layers of the population.

Often an excessive burdening, that the person's strength cannot cope with, leads to various forms of mistreatment. Anyone can get into such situations. The following experiment was recorded on video: A woman was locked up together with a constantly crying child. She could not get out, and became more and more desperate. After 24 hours she was so desperate that she wanted to suffocate the child with a pillow. Conclusion: Everyone is at risk if the burden exceeds the withstanding capacity.

Risk factors

1. People who have been mistreated in their childhood and adolescence tend themselves again to mistreat children.
2. Adopted children, disabled children, premature births are more vulnerable.
3. The social situation of the family – being a single parent, financial hardship, housing that is too small, etc. – can encourage mistreatment.
4. Certain beliefs like, for instance, a dogmatic religiosity, can lead to overly strict up-bringing.
5. Young immature parents do not come up with adequate reactions to their children's behavior due to their educational inability.

Children challenge us! They push us to our limits because they want to get to know them. Parents learn from children. When a child – consciously or unconsciously – is mistreated and then is not consoled, the adult violates the integrity of the child – his ego-development is obstructed. The actual task of the parents and also the educator and caregiver is, to ask themselves: What does this child need now at this age so that he can fulfill his earthly tasks?

In the last years we could observe that the healthy intuition, that is, the immediate knowledge of what is right for the development dwindled more and more. In the time of the consciousness soul it is the task of Waldorf schools, kindergartens, and doctors, to offer help to parents, to advise them, and to strengthen them in their good intentions, also to prevent mistreatment.

Symptoms of mistreatment of the infant

- The child is thin, malnourished, transparent; has bruises, frequent injuries.
- The child cramps and stiffens when touched – during diapering, also when examined by the doctor.
- Hospitalism: rocking, no eye contact, a tendency to retreat – these are signs of incarnation difficulties, brought on by outer trauma.
- The child never cries or always cries.
- Shrill screaming.
- Refusing to eat or eats greedily.
- Mold infections or redness in the genital area can – but must not at this age – generate suspicion (but certainly later).
- Bladder infection. Examination of the diaper or urine of sperm is necessary.
- Sleeping problems, sleep disturbances, night mares.
- Frequent infections can be an indication of not being treated well or not being well incarnated.
- Strong, unexplainable pains (head, stomach), accompanied by frequent or excessive dispensing of pain medication.
- Munchhausensymptom: The child is purposely made ill through medication or something other. The mother (other persons) then receives a form of recognition, when she visits a doctor or goes to the hospital. Many, often stationary examinations are necessary to find out the real reasons. (Question of self-medication?)

of the young child/toddler

- The child is not brought to the group regularly; the child is only seen by the doctor at long intervals; the parents tell different stories at different places concerning the causes.
- The child does not laugh at all or cries constantly, he clings to the care person and does not want to be cared for by someone else.
- The child «flows out» into the environment; when contact is made, he scratches, bites, hits, tickles, cannot set limits to his behavior.
- The child turns his attention again and again to the genitals and touches them – either his own or those of other children or adults.
- Very hesitant when going to the toilet.
- Isolation of the children: The child is not allowed to play with others, may not go into their homes, may not participate in certain things in the group, i.e. swimming, or any sports.
- The child orients himself very much on his siblings.
- Defecation.
- Bed wetting and wetting during the day. (You have to wonder how far the ego development has progressed. Is it a constitutional question? Bedwetting during the night certainly has other causes than wetting during the day.)
- Self-destruction.

- Lack of containment. Child always wants to lie down.

Further Symptoms
- Significant change in the «physical» expression.
- The children strongly assert themselves outwardly, above all boys, or pull back very strongly, especially the girls.
- The drawings of the children can be very revealing. Often something is missing or the genitals can be seen in the picture. A predominance of black on the picture or framing his/her own figure, are expressions of deep loneliness.
- The children do not want to be in a circle with the group; they do not want to be looked at.
- They do not want to be dressed or undressed.
- When walking they pinch together buttocks and thighs.
- The children either come to school very early or always too late.
- The children never tell anything about their home in the group.
- The affected families move a lot, change doctors and therapists a lot.
- The children always say the same thing, for instance, «Daddy broke a banana last night».
- Mixed food arouses disgust.
- The children chew on sleeves or pants etc.
- They exaggerate in terms of personal hygiene, e.g. they often wash their hands.
- The parents are anxious to draw a picture of perfection, are also helpful. In conversation, the problem is reduced to the kindergarten – as educator, guilt feelings arise: At home, there seems to be no problems.
- The child is always the victim.
- The child always stays in the corners of the schoolyard or seeks closeness the teacher.

An example from the practice:
A mother comes into the office with a child with asthma. She complains, cries, is absolutely helpless. The child puts her hand on her mother's lap and says: «Everything will be alright!» It is noticeable that the child is protecting the mother.

Basic questions
When we perceive the symptoms, the tragedy has already happened – we are always too late for abuse and mistreatment. That is why we usually have guilt feelings and reproach ourselves that we did not notice the child's suffering and did not intervene immediately.

A further dilemma is, that the listed symptoms can also point to other illnesses or disturbances or may reveal certain dispositions.

When do they clearly indicate abuse or mistreatment?

All of us – doctors, educators, nurses, therapists, teachers, day-mothers, children's group leaders, etc. – should be familiar with the symptoms of abuse, mistreatment and neglect, we should be alert. Since there are also other causes for almost all symptoms, we must train our awareness, for the etheric that is also affected by abuse. We should gather our observations and communicate with one another as objectively as possible to verify them. If e.g. several people observe the child's movements over a longer period of time and have an exchange with one another, thus creating a picture of the child which would lead to further understanding. It is necessary to focus on the phenomena, let them speak and then, in a conversation come to clarity of the circumstances. Then the first steps for a healing can be taken.

But there should not be created any negative mood that could be transferred to other children. Many situations are pedagogically less than optimal and require a high degree of patience and compassionate love.

What does abuse have to do with karma?
There are human beings who fit together well, and humans who do not fit together; and yet, they have something in common: They cannot let go of one another. Hate and love are very close – also perpetrators and victims. Usually the karmic relationship between perpetrator and victim (child) remains hidden; we may only assume that there is a connection. For both it is important that the perpetrator comes to his senses during his life and tries to clarify the relationship with his victim.

Effects of abuse on the members of the human organization

– Ether-body and abuse of the physical

In physical, that is, in sexual abuse, the physical body of the child is damaged. If someone is traumatized, according to Rudolf Steiner, the connection of the etheric body is loosened from the physical. When the trauma recurs, part of the etheric body constantly remains outside; an «etheric island» is formed by the etheric body. The child then has a «hole» in his etheric body.

With constant abuse the perpetrator and the victim (child) form a common ether body – as is also the case when people regularly undertake something together with others, e.g. in work-groups, groups of the Anthroposophic Society, in the conferences with teachers and educators, etc. Since the ether body is the seat of our habit life, the child cannot do anything else but take on the habits of the perpetrator. Even when the abuse comes to an end, the hole in the child's ether body remains. That is also the reason why children and adults who were abused for a longer period of time, succumb so quickly to abuse by others. The hole in the ether body «sucks in» the ether body of the other, and the person loses his independent decision making power.

– Etheric and soul mistreatment

Inadequate provision of food, clothing, hygiene, the absence of parental love, etc. is actually a mistreatment of the etheric. For the daily, regular providing affects the etheric body – it is damaged by the deficiency.

By psychic abuse, the astral sensation and -expansion of the child is paralyzed; they are replaced by the astral wishes of the parents: Too much responsibility is burdened on the children, or they are treated too long as a little child; they have to take up hobbies of the parents, only because they want it, while s/he has no inclination towards it. This causes damage to the astral body. If this is accompanied by trauma and an etheric island has already been formed, corresponding «astral islands» can form that show themselves in the form of fixed ideas and/or compulsive feelings.

– Splitting of the I – the multiple personality disorder

In the worst case, multiple personality disorders can occur, in which everything that the astral body experiences can no longer be held together by the ego: when a child is traumatized, s/he tries to protect her/himself by pulling herself out of the action with her ego. If s/he experiences the violence too often, the ego also forms an «island». It separates off from the everyday self which continues to evolve. If the traumatization continues, more and more parts of the ego separate. Finally, multiple personalities live in the I/ego, e.g., the wife, the mother, the prostitute, the bar-tender, the little child. The peculiar thing is, that the one does not know about the others. The aspects of the soul that we hold together with the help of our I become separated in the multiple personality disorder.

– Guilt feelings in children

The Nigerian author Buchi Emecheta describes in her book Gwendolin[1], how a girl that lives with her grandmother is raped numerous times by a friend of the family. She finally speaks about this to the family. The «uncle» is expelled from the village community. But after a few months the grandmother complains that she does not have enough to eat anymore because the «uncle» does not come anymore. Later Gwendolin goes to her parents in London. When her mother goes back to her grandmother, the father assaults the girl. She is afraid to talk about it. He is her dear father! If he is not around, who will care for the younger sister and brothers? Also, in England such a father goes to prison. Buchi Emecheta describes the whole story that we sympathize how first of all, the child is silenced and second, feels that she herself is the guilty one.

– How do guilt feelings develop?

If I have an ideal image of how something should be, and do not have the strength to endure the fact that I cannot reach the ideal, I feel insecure, something starts to «wobble». I feel guilty. Debt is always a negative account. An ideal too lofty, brings us into the realm of Lucifer, and if we cannot reach the ideal, then we fall into Ahriman's realm – into the realm of guilt-(feelings).

The adult represents a natural authority for the child; he seems like a divine being. When the adult does something that does not correspond with that oversized picture, the child cannot process that experience, not digest it; she plunges deeply into feelings of guilt.

---

[1] Buchi Emecheta, *Gwendolin*. In: *Töchter Afrikas*. 2. ed. München 1998.

Basics for the therapy of abuse

If a trauma has occurred, a rehabilitation therapy for the etheric body or others of the subtle members of the human organization, must be initiated as soon as possible. For this reason, Rudolf Steiner's pedagogical and curative basic laws are essential, as presented in the Curative Education Course[2] the therapist must know, that his higher member works on the next lower member of the organization of the child in a healing way:

- The ether body of the educator/therapist works in a healing way on the physical body of the child.
- The astral body of the educator/therapist works in a healing way on the ether body of the child.
- The I of the educator/therapist works in a healing way on the astral body of the child.
- The spirit-self of the educator/therapist works in a healing way on the I of the child.

Since we have not yet developed the spirit-self in our present time, we are not able as individuals to heal the consequences of abuse. This requires the intensive cooperation of several people; then a spirit-self is formed by working together in a cooperative way.

However, if I alone am responsible for a patient, whose I is not yet available, I turn to the guardian angel of the patient and ask him to help and work together with me. We cannot heal «against karma». We are also never able to eliminate all pain or heal all illnesses.

Anthroposophic trauma therapy

With the help of anthroposophic medicaments and outer applications by an anthroposophic doctor, it is possible to «lure back» the ether body that was loosened from the physical by trauma. Through outer applications the person's organ of touch that is spread over the whole body, is addressed – then the ether body becomes interested again in the physical body. This therapy has to be applied with a great feeling of tact. Conversations with the doctor or therapist (psychologist) are necessary, and can help the patient that s/he can manage to tell the whole story, to process and digest it. For a child play therapy is more useful.

If the traumatization has far advanced or if the event was in the far past so that the astral body has formed islands, then in addition psychotherapy is needed, often also art therapy. Biography work can also be helpful: The trauma is seen in connection with the whole life, and this makes it easier to speak about it and work on it. Through this work the trauma loses the power that it often exerts on the whole life, so that the beautiful moments of life, that were before as if darkened, can begin to shine again. In the art therapy one can often see months before the patient can put the event into words, where the threat came from.

The deeply rooted guilt feelings and fixed ideas that are attached to the etheric islands, bring the person every day into

---

2 Rudolf Steiner, *Curative Education*. GA 317.

unwanted situations. I ask the patient to imagine such a situation and then paint as detailed a picture as possible. At my suggestion, she is to think of help for this situation. In this way, I have stimulated his/her will and somewhat mitigated the compulsion.

When it is about abuse, about the sphere of the I, we need to work together, not only in the therapeutic facility, but also with the schools, child psychiatrists, pediatricians, family assistance, educational counselling centers, advice centers on abuse issues, and so on. It is worthwhile to seek information and advice in counseling centers.

Prevention of further abuse
If there is a reasonable suspicion of abuse, special attention must be paid to a few situations:
- In kindergarten, one should not let the affected children go to the toilet alone, especially if there are also older children.
- When a «beautiful little house» of cloths and furniture is created, every 5 to 10 minutes an educator should come «for a visit» and look around.

Hanne Looij
The Madonna as source of strength

1. The Madonna as source of strength for the body

How can art, especially a Madonna picture, be a help when caring for our health?

Rudolf Steiner pointed out, that perceiving is not a passive reacting to impressions that leave their traces in form of an image, imprint or projection in our eye or in another sense organ. Perception is much more an activity in which the whole person is involved. When we consciously perceive something, we imitate it inwardly; this process is not about reflection without will, but about new, personal creation.

When we look at a picture, the etheric body starts to move in a certain way, depending on the colors and shapes that we perceive. The etheric body reproduces the movements and forms of the composition and the gestures of the figures – actually also the color and form of the room in which we are. If we are not clairvoyant, this process happens subconsciously.[1]

This way, we understand that the regular viewing of a Madonna picture can have a healing and soothing effect on us; it helps to bring the etheric streams into balance and harmony. The Madonna pictures by Raffael are particularly suitable for this, especially the so-called Madonna picture series, which the physician Felix Peipers put together in 1911 in collaboration with Rudolf Steiner. These individual pictures should be viewed in a specific order.[2]

For the picture sequence, placement and movement of the child in relation to the mother is decisive: The child stands on the earth by her right or left leg; he is carried on one arm or the other; and the foreheads of mother and child touch, and so on. The sequence is chosen that the child, in relation to the body of the mother describes the figure of a pentagram. The series begins with the Sixtine Madonna where the whole composition is strongly shaped by the pentagram and ends with a detail from the transfiguration of Christ, where the figure of Christ also forms a pentagram.

If you look at the whole series and participate in the movement of the child with respect to the mother, you notice that the pictures themselves are only like stations on the path and that the actual movement takes place between the pictures. The movement itself is not visible. We owe it to our etheric body that we can still follow it in the invisible.

If we immerse ourselves meditatively in this series of Madonna pictures, the different streams of our ether body are stimulated in a healing way. If this exercise is done before going to sleep, it strengthens the affect further. It is very suitable for expectant mothers but also for people with heart problems and sleep-disturbances or fears.[3]

---

1 Rudolf Steiner, *Rosicrucianism Renewed – the Unity of Art, Science and Religion*. GA 284, Lecture on 15. October 1911, evening.
2 Edited by Robert R. Nuber: *Die heilende Madonnenbildreihe nach Felix Peipers und Rudolf Steiner*. Stuttgart 1997 *(the healing series of Madonna pictures from Felix Peipers and Rudolf Steiner)*.
3 Walther Bühler geht tiefer auf die heilende Wirkung der Übung ein und beschreibt sehr schön, wie die Aktivität des Ätherleibes mit dem Inhalt der Bilder übereinstimmt: *Die meditative Madonnenbildserie*. Novalis, Nr. 12, 1, 1993/94. *(Series of meditative Madonnas).*

2. The Madonna as a source of strength for the soul

What can this archetypal picture of mother and child teach the care giver and educator concerning our inner conduct towards the child?

For this aspect, we looked at the Maria in the Rosenhag, which Stefan Lochner painted in Cologne between the years 1447 and 1450, towards the end of his life.

The mentioned picture is quite small (40 x 50 cm), so it is probably meant for the viewer to establish a very personal relationship to the illustrated figures. It is painted very lovingly and to the finest detail, apparently with a one- or two-haired brush.

In the middle sits Mary with the child in her lap. Her deep blue robe spreads in many folds across a red cushion and across small green plants. On her head she wears a richly decorated crown and a precious brooch on her breast. In a circle open to the front but around them, are many small angels making music, folding their hands and handing out either a rose or an apple. They wear red, blue and yellow robes. Behind Maria an arbor is recognizable on which grow red and white roses. – The background is golden and interspersed with many fine rays, all emanating from a golden semicircle. From this semicircle a gracious old man is looking down on Mary. Between his protective hands, a white dove is about to descend. Around him are many little angelic heads. And in the right and left upper corner you can see angels holding open a richly decorated red curtain.

The picture is strongly symmetrical. Only the child falls out of symmetry. This is offset by the slight inclination of Mary's head and the gesture of her right hand.

The horizontal structure is thus determined by a duality: Below, the green of the meadow dominates with the many plants; everything shines in gold above. Both areas are connected by the figure of Mary and by the arbor. The figure of Mary with the mantle forms an equilateral triangle; a second inverted triangle is formed by the lines in the arbor. Both triangles interpenetrate – Mary's head is at the point of the intersection. At the intersection of the imaginary diagonals is the brooch.

What can this picture tell us about Mary and her relationship to the child?

The symmetry of the composition with the two triangles causes great stillness and balance in the picture. This impression is reinforced by the deep blue of the robe and the introspective gaze of Mary. The amulet plays a major role in the composition: The eye of the beholder is attracted by it and then comes to rest. We can experience this point as inner center of Mary, as source of her inner peace. And this experience communicates itself to our own body, that we perceive our own heart as inner center.

Mary is at home in two worlds and at the same time represents the connection between these worlds: she sits humbly in the living green of the earth; the upper body and the head, however, rise in a royal attitude into the gold of the sky. On the one hand, she is strongly connected to the earth; on the other hand, she finds her

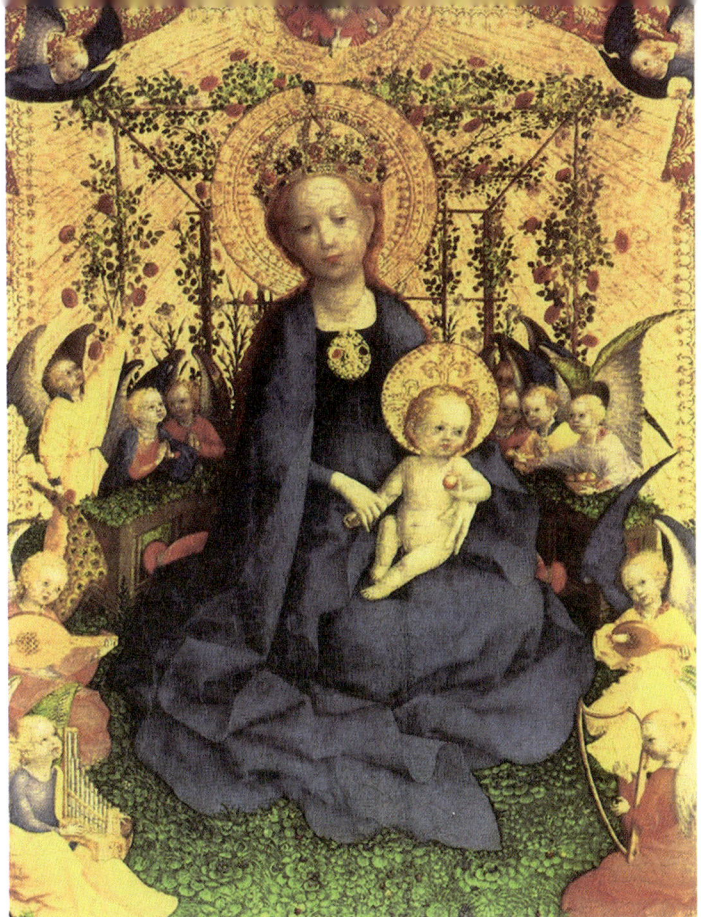

Fig. 1: Stefan Lochner, Maria im Rosenhag. Wallraf-Richartz-Museum, Köln

strength in the heavens open to her. In between, roses grow – as an image of her soul, which strives to rise to the spiritual. The roses are rooted firmly in the earth, and the woody branches bear hard, painful thorns. But from this death-related realm rise noble, delicate, fragrant flowers. This process of becoming ever more noble and pure is completed in the crown, where the earthly flowers have become heavenly flowers of precious stones.

Numerous angels form a protective semicircle around mother and child and create a space of security. It is demarcated toward the outside and yet open; the viewer feels invited to join the circle himself. – The same gesture can be found on the coat: Protective and demarcated, it rests on the shoulders, but also leaves room for the meeting with the child. – And for a third time the same gesture appears – in the hands of Mary: they support, guide, accompany, «feel the pulse of the child», but also leave him free. Nowhere is there coercion or pressuring will.

The child occupies a special position in the picture. He is the only figure in the picture that is naked. He shows himself unveiled, as it is, in his innocence, purity and vulnerability. By breaking the symmetry, he brings life and movement into the composition. Through the gestures of the hands and the head of the mother, the balance is restored. – The child looks to the right and beyond the picture. Right is the side where we are active, the side where we experience the future. In this picture it is also the side where the light comes from; on the left are shadows. Also, as far as the gaze is concerned, the mother restores the balance, in that she turns the head in the opposite direction and looks more inward. – The child is seated but makes an active impression. With the opened, bent little legs he shows the intention to move, while the mother sits in complete calmness.

Even when we do not take into account the medieval symbolic – God Father, Holy Spirit, the apple of paradise, red and white roses, white lilies, the many small plants in the green –, the picture alone through its composition, the colors, the light shows us how new life can arise, when heaven and earth touch, and when we consciously strive to lift the earth to the heavens and to embed the spirit in the earth. This connection creates a kind of center in which a great peace can be experienced. And this calmness enables a renewing, living movement. Looking inward is a condition for looking outward into a future. The pure higher Self can only show itself, when it can live is a space of warmth and security; and a free space can only develop where limits are set.

The two angels above hold the curtain open for us, so that we can see something that is normally hidden. In the process of perception, we lift the veil ourselves: We bring to our consciousness, the effect of the colors and forms on our soul – an effect that shows itself also by a fleeting observation, but then remains below the threshold of consciousness.

3. The Madonna as source of strength for the spirit

What can the pictures of Mary tell us about our relationship with the spiritual world?

In a lecture about «Isis and Madonna» Rudolf Steiner[4], relates how we can see in the Madonna a picture for the human soul, that has purified itself of all that pulls it to the sensual, and chains thinking to the physical body. Through the catharsis, the soul, the spiritual eye can awaken and give birth to the human being's higher I. When the human soul (Mary) opens itself to the spirit and takes it (the father) in, then the soul can awaken the spirit within (the Son).

We could see the life of Mary as a reflection of the development of the human soul. The different steps of maturity in her life reflect the evolution of consciousness of humanity.

There are two occurrences in her life where she experiences directly the Holy Spirit: The Annunciation and the outpouring of the Holy Spirit at Pentecost.

Two pictures follow, on which these two events are presented: one originating around 1400, an Annunciation, and a Pentecost presentation from the 12th century (see Fig. 2 and 3 on the following pages).

From the composition as well as from the posture and the gestures we can «read» the inner attitude and condition

---

[4] Rudolf Steiner, *Where and How does one Find the Spirit?* GA 57, Rudolf Steiner Archiv 2015, lecture of 29. April 1909, *Isis and Madonna*. Dornach 1984.

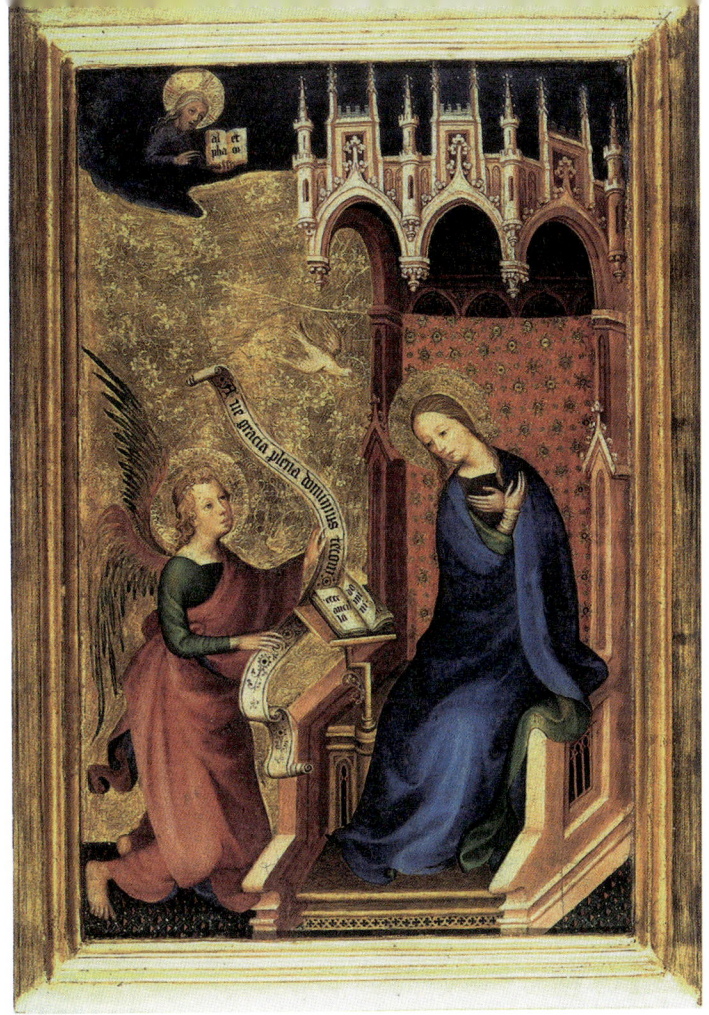

Fig. 2: Unknown painter, Annunciation, from a travel-altar. The Walters Art Gallery, Baltimore

under which Maria approaches the spiritual world. She can become a model for our own spiritual life and spiritual development:

Annunciation: Mary experiences the effect of the Holy Spirit during an encounter with an angel.

Pentecost: Mary experiences the effect of the Holy Spirit when she is together with twelve people, who are experiencing the same.

Annunciation: Mary and the angel both occupy half of the picture.

Pentecost: Mary is in the middle, the largest, meaning, most important figure in the group.

Annunciation: Mary is deeply moved, her body is bending. She reacts with feeling.

Pentecost: Mary is very up-right, a frontal view. She reacts from her I.

Annunciation: Mary has her arms crossed and looks inward. She is full of humility and would like to retreat.

Pentecost: Mary has her hands in an open gesture. Her gaze is awake and

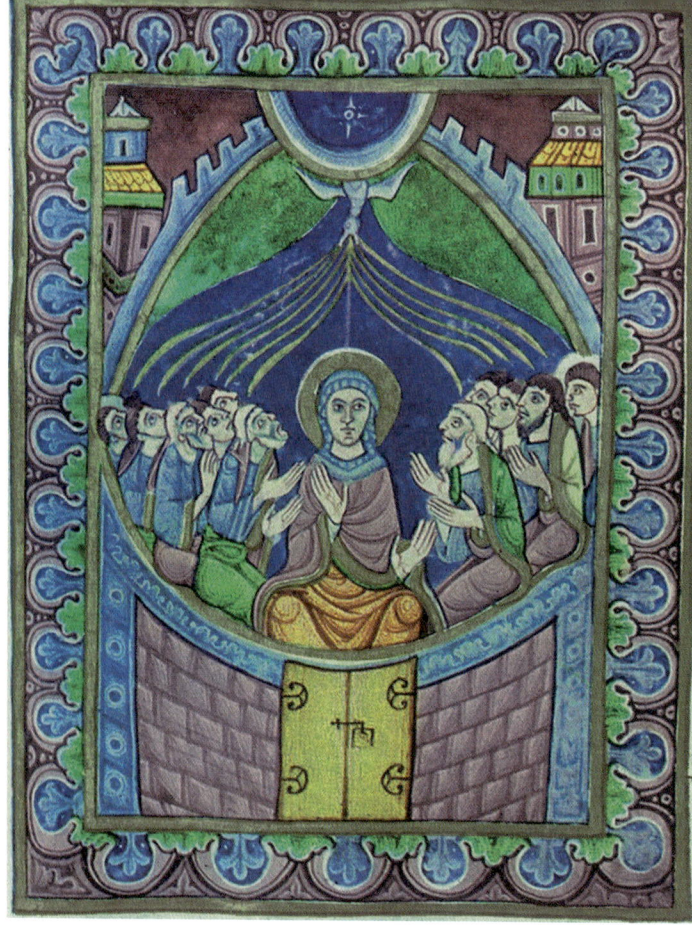

Fig. 3: Pentecost, Psalter from St Alban Abbey near London, 12th century. Hildesheim. St. Godehard Kunstverlag, D-56653 Maria Laach, Card nr. 5672

«all-seeing». She takes up her space consciously and completely.

Annunciation: Mary is taking in, listening and completely with the angel.

Pentecost: Mary is receiving. She is consciously opening herself, in listening she is awake, very concentrated and in inner balance.

Annunciation: Mary has a roof above her; the room is open to the side.

Pentecost: Mary is in a closed room; upwards, i.e. inward, an area that is beyond space and is completely open, is forming.

Annunciation: The dove is flying diagonally to Mary.

Pentecost: The dove is vertically above Mary.

Annunciation: The rays come from the mouth of Christ; the dove flies in the rays.

Pentecost: The rays come from the beak of the dove and aim to the heads of the individual human beings. The dove is connected to a semicircle in which there is a kind of star or eye.

We see how Mary, a young, pure, «white» girl, gifted with, as well as surprised by, an encounter with a supersensible being, develops into a fully conscious woman, who is now able out of the power of a human community in which every individual is inwardly active, to create a direct and fully awake connection with the Holy Spirit. In her youth she shows her openness as readiness to take on her fate. At the end of her life, after she experienced and suffered her destiny intensely, she opens herself out of her acquired wisdom in order to establish a conscious connection with the spirit.

There seems to be a deeper reason, that Rudolf Steiner comes to speak about the picture of the Sistine Madonna at the opening of the Stuttgart building.[5] For the image of the Madonna is deeply connected with the task of Anthroposophy. It shows us, that out of the human soul the higher I of man can be born, how the human being receives his life-impulses from the spiritual world, and how he can give them a physical «body», by realizing his innermost impulses on earth. The picture of the Madonna thus makes us recognize the process of knowledge itself as the birth process. When we delve into the pictures of the Madonna actively, they do not remain outside of us, but they connect with us and help our soul to become more and more sensitive and open, so that it can experience these thoughts as spiritual reality. Madonna pictures make our soul capable of birth. I hope that the Madonna pictures will always find their way to children, the parents and educators, into group rooms and bedrooms, for parents' evenings and to educational consultations, to meetings of the faculty, the playgroup or day care facility – and just for meditation.

---

[5] Rudolf Steiner, *Rosicrucianism Renewed – the Unity of Art, Science and Religion*. GA 284, Lecture on 15. October 1911, evening.

Brigitte Huisinga
Parent-Child-Groups

What are parents looking for with their very young children in parent-child-groups, and what can we offer them?

The current situation of young parents

Parent-child groups from baby age onward are the trend. There is hardly a mother who does not inquire, sometimes already before the birth of her child, what she can do with her baby, such as a baby massage, baby swimming, crawling groups, PEKiP (Prague Parent-Child Program). Parents want to do the best for their child; at the same time the changed life situations bring about new needs and necessities.

The care and education of young children no longer naturally follows traditional practices. The societally conditioned isolation on the one hand, and on the other the great flood of information with regard to all that is necessary and important for young children in order to be able to stand strong later on in the battle of competition. These shape the relationship between parent and child from the beginning.

Many questions from parents revolve around the development of their child, but they are also asking for suggestions concerning the necessary assistance.

How much care does my child need?
How much sleep?
What should I play with him?

The changed life situation is reflected in the following statement by a mother: «I always wanted a family. Now I have two small children and a husband who leaves the house at eight in the morning; and does not return before seven in the evening. He is working. My days revolve around the children and the household. I do not work. I have vacation. Child raising vacation. But I do not feel relaxed, but alone, often stressed, overwhelmed and overburdened!»

Expectations and reality do not coincide. One's own role must be redefined, including the right balance between the needs of the child and one's own.

Different educational institutions are taking up the situation of young parents. Confessional Family Education Centers offer a comprehensive program for birth preparation, baby massage, etc. The numerous groups for parents and children beginning at about 5 months to kindergarten age, offer above all contact with other parents which means exchange and mutual support, and for the children play and fun. – Also groups in Mother-centers, that build on the personal initiative of the members and make available primarily exchange with one another and activity with the child.

With baby-swimming as well as baby-massage and the groups that work according to the Parent-Child Program (PEKiP), there are additional remedial aspects which require a special training of group leaders.

Parent-child groups as part of Waldorf education

How do parent-child-groups need to be designed that primarily want to safeguard the dignity of the young child?

The precondition is, that we recognize the group work with parents and children from baby age onward as a necessary component of parenting work. At the same time, we should create conditions that are appropriate for the young child and for the parents with their demands and questions so that they are not prevented from accessing us. The question is:

> *How does the anthroposophic picture of the human being come to life in the course of group work and also in the outer design?*

In the following, work with parent-child groups in the free educational institution «der hof» in Niederursel, is described as an example. The parent-child-group-work here has a long-standing tradition. So, above all, we try to create space in a comprehensive sense – a space into which, first of all, calmness can enter, in which nobody «has to», in which all tension and expectation falls away; a space where respect, warmth and consideration as well as trust in the development of the child and the ability of the parents, come into being. In this space, we want to give the parents the possibility to perceive their child in such a way, that this perceiving will help them to come to their own solutions and understanding. The group leader must know the development of the young child very well, in order to give help in this process of perceiving.

Assessing the development of movement correctly

The movement development of babies varies much. It may be that one child of the group crawls already at the age of seven months, another at this age still lies contentedly on his back and plays intensely with his hands and feet and handles objects, that he himself was able to reach when lying on his side. The parents of the second child are often exposed to the commentaries by the surrounding world, whether the pace of their child's development is still sufficient. As a leading care person of the group, you have to know that the development of movement can differ up to the age of 6 months – one child learns to walk at 11 months, the other not till 19 months – but she also has to be able to see:

- whether the fine motor development is age-appropriate
- whether the child is interested, whether she perceives
- whether mother and child are in contact
- whether development is slowly progressing.

A parent-child group has a familiar atmosphere in which every mother and every child has the feeling: Here I am at the right place. Competition or mutual peer review have no place. For every mother, her child is the dearest and most beautiful. It is especially useful for the very little ones to move from mother and child to mother and child and give each couple a little attention individually, to look at the child with joy and just to see what s/he is doing.

Age-appropriate development

A comprehensive knowledge of the nature and development of children is important because, depending on the age of the children, the environment and the course of group lessons must differ. For babies, a song at the beginning, accompanied by the children's harp, and a song at the end. Orientation: «Now I am here again» or «Now we will go home again into our familiar environment.» Later a brief ending can be added with a seasonal hand-gesture game. We should always pay attention that the repetition is a joy for the children and not a principle that we follow. We need to sense constantly how much is right for this group of children.

The leading care person of the group makes sure that the materials for their play are fitting to the development of the children. She also knows how to arrange these in an appealing way, so that the children feel invited to take them, and that the parents get ideas for the play environment at home.

Movement offers must not be dangerous to any child or call forth the anxiety of the parents. On the other hand, the children need and seek appropriate adventures. It is the task to accompany the children well, and when you have fearful parents, to be close to the children when they try something new, and to assist them in such a way that the trust of the parents grows in the ability and personal initiative of the children.

In addition to the weekly group lessons with the young children, there are regular parent evenings, where the mothers and fathers have the opportunity to speak in more detail and to ask questions. Also, here perceptions and wishes concerning the group lessons are exchanged.

Public theme evenings
Furthermore, public and overarching themes for all groups are offered, such as:
- how parents can accompany their child on the way to independent eating
- how a child develops from lying down to walking
- topics and questions about everyday life with young children.

In the parent evenings and theme evenings, we try to make the world of the small child comprehensible to the parents using our own experiences.

An example: Various familiar things are shown. The participants immediately verify them with a concept. The more unknown a displayed object is, the more it is explored with the senses, the more similar it is to a child's approach. It is felt, tapped, listened, smelled or tasted. While we as adults are subject to goal-oriented thinking and speed, the child still delves into things and in that process, experiences himself.

Such tangible examples can provide parents with understanding and new perspectives on their child's development and behavior.

Parents weeks
Another option for continuing to learn to be a parent, are the «parents' weeks», happening once a year. We consider the development of the child on the basis of anthroposophic knowledge of the human being, and try to work with it in an understandable and descriptive way.

This very brief report on our work with parent-child groups at the «hof» may give an idea of the amount of qualification and background knowledge necessary to help parents and children in group work: Beyond the study of anthroposophic knowledge of the human being, it is necessary that the group leadership has experience to deal with group processes, conflicts and modern methods of adult education. Last but not least, it is important to be willing to reflect on oneself in order to avoid transfers and projections. Then the parent-child group can become a true-to-life learning field for educational content and child-friendly behavior for all those involved.

May this insight into our work inspire you to have your own ideas and to have courage, to develop something new according to the respective conditions.

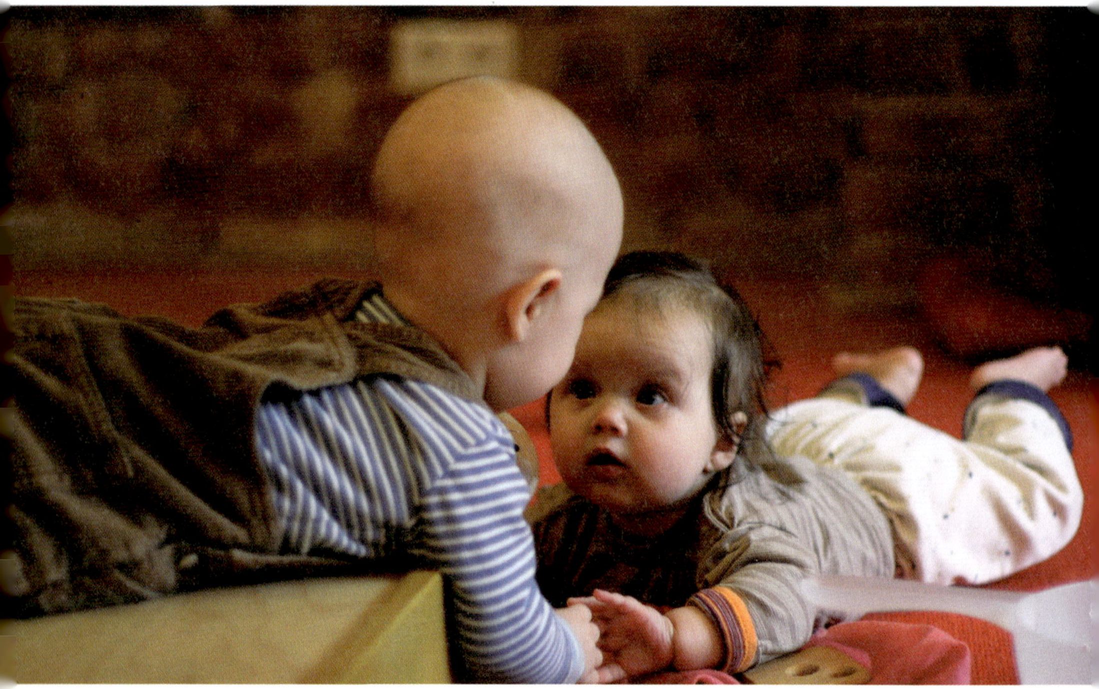

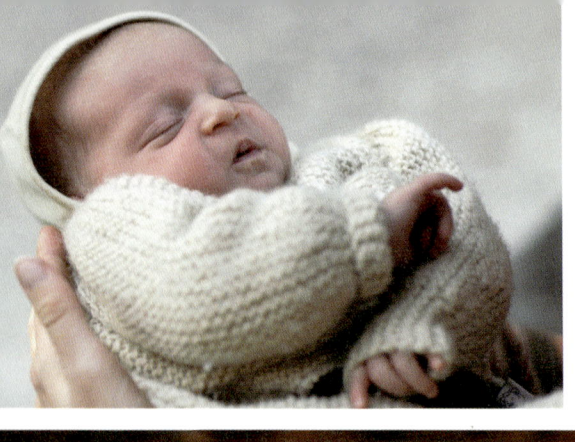
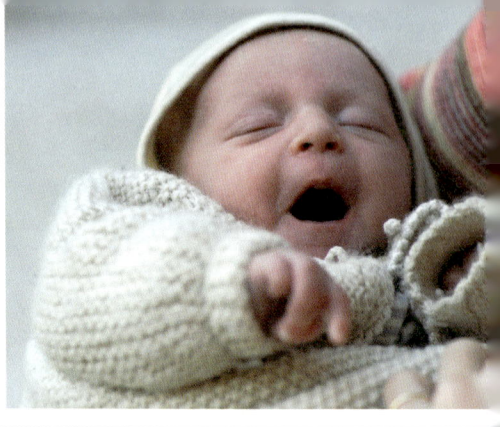
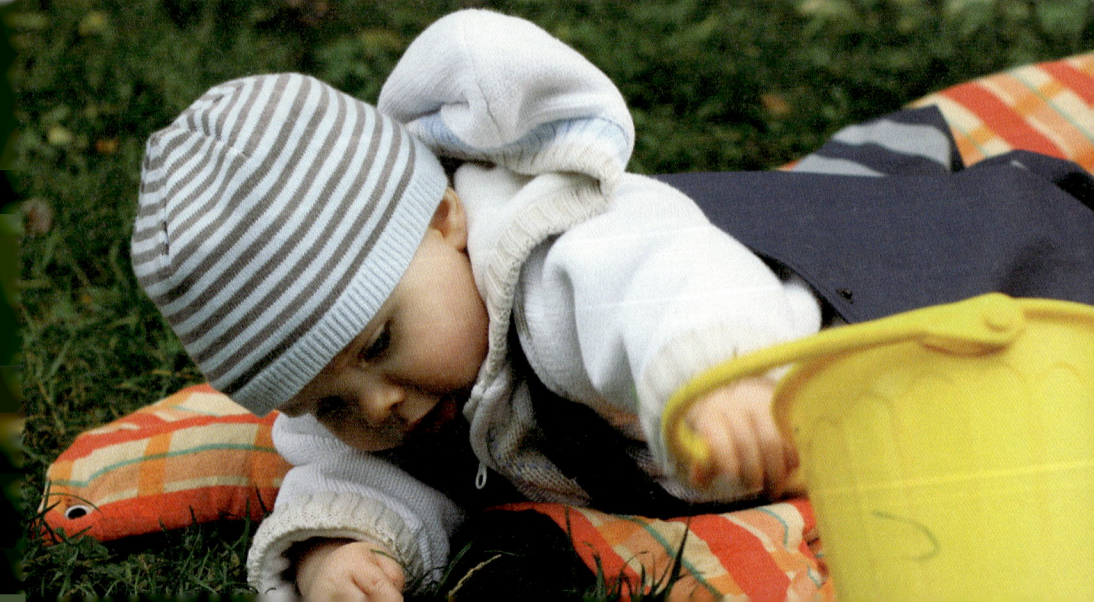

The working group on the young child (AKK)
Quality indicators for centers catering for the young child

1. Preamble

Far reaching social changes have occurred in recent years. They have to do with changes in the way women are perceived and how couples relate, with the decline in birth rates and the consequences for the labor market. These have a serious effect on family structures. The challenge of those engaged with Waldorf education is to find ways of ensuring in their institutions that despite these changes, childhood is given the protection it needs.

The conferences on «The dignity of the small child» that were held in Dornach in 2000, Järna in 2004 and Dornach in 2010, gave rise to many ideas. These crystallized around the need to develop a further training concept for those caring for infants and small children that is based on Rudolf Steiner's understanding of the human being.

The first three years are very important for a person's whole life and it is vital that a heightened awareness is focused on them. The needs of the young child and the results of research into early childhood development must be taken into account and then put into practice.

AKK Kleinkind (working group on the young child)
The working group «Arbeitskreis Kleinkind (AKK)», made up of teachers who carry out active research in training centres and in their daily work, has worked together to develop quality indicators that can give guidance to those working with young children in Waldorf inspired centres.

Structuring the living and working area
The educational concept underpinning a centre needs to ensure that the spatial and temporal structure of the care reflects the elementary needs and developmental requirements of the small child in the best possible way. These include the following essential conditions:

– **Security and Connectedness:**
Reliable person to relate to, careful acclimatization, transparent procedures in the day, reliable spatial structures, time for building a care relationship.

An additional area for providing care in the group room is necessary in order to make the caring activity of the adult visible to all children.

– **Discovery and Exploration:**
Prepared surroundings, sufficient space and opportunity for movement and play both indoors and outside; adequate range of stimulating, age appropriate play things.

– **Caring for the surroundings:**
This point is about care, food, choice of toys and materials and how the space is arranged.

– **Experience of one's own activity:**
Meeting the previously mentioned conditions allows the children to experience the effect of their own activity. In the plan of the day they must be given sufficient space and time to develop autonomy and independence (to help with the work, at meal times etc.).

2. Qualification of the co-worker – foundation in Waldorf education

The basic pre-condition is the state recognition of the educator or such equivalent recognition of a classroom helper as may be legally determined. The additional Waldorf teaching qualification of those engaged is recommended.

What is essential in every case however is a further qualification in the anthroposophical approach to the education of small children.

Requirements of co-workers
- A study of the anthroposophical understanding of the human being with a special emphasis on «pre-birth existence» and on the first three years of life.
- Biography work: In order to attain a professional attitude as an educator it is vital to gain an understanding of one's own development and one's own physical and psychological health.
- Willingness to work together with parents, colleagues, trustees of the institution, the region.
- Willingness to undergo supervision and advisory discussions with colleagues (inter vision) as well as continual professional development and further training.

Accepting children under three years
- To take children under three years of age requires the agreement of the entire colleague group and the trustees of the Kindergarten or school. It can only be successful if work with the small child is accepted and carried by the whole community.
- The importance and value of bearing joint responsibility in an educational partnership is paramount. Part of this is acceptance of the family situation.
- The concept document must include the working practices of the institution.
- The acclimatization phase needs very careful planning and forms part of the described concept document.
- The importance of having a person to relate to in the institution must be recognized and acknowledged in any replacement plan (firm, trusted replacements).

3. Institutional framework

The framework should take account of:
- the teacher – child relationship (staffing)
- the size of the group
- the qualifications of the teaching staff.

The time of preparation and clearing up as well as professional development and further training of the teaching staff, the spatial and material equipping of the centre as well as the ongoing educational and care work.

Differing national and regional regulations need to be taken into account (see «Standards for institutional frameworks in Kindergarten centres – Professional assessment of the German welfare federation»).

Mixed age groups from 2 to 6 years
- **Maximum 15 children,** with a maximum of 5 children under 3 years old. Staff-child ratio: 2:15 and one assistant, student on work experience.

- **Individually tailored content:** Agree a plan for the day that reflects the needs of children in their differing stages of development.
- **Special room design concept:** Sufficient space for both younger and older children, dedicated play and movement areas that can be separated off.
- **Care facilities** in the secure infant play area, quiet room, age appropriate toys.
- **Acclimatization plan**

If the above conditions cannot be achieved this kind of group structure is not recommended.

Groups with children aged between 1 and 3 years
- **Maximum 10 children**

Staff-child ratio: 2:10 plus an assistant. To prepare for the transition into Kindergarten regular contact with the Kindergarten should be encouraged.

Groups with children aged between 0 and 3 years
- **Maximum 10 children**

Staff-child ratio: 1:3, maximum 1:4. The above recommendations apply here too.

– Additional considerations:

No more than 10 children should be accepted in these groups. It has been found helpful for such mixed age groups to be split into two groups of those aged between 0 and 1½ and between 1½ and 3 years old.

It is a good idea to have a separate play area for children who are still crawling.

Resource addresses

Martin Plackner
Alkersdorf 21, A-4880 St. Georgen
Tel. 0043/7667/8662
www.spielzeugmacher.at
high chairs for meal times, climbing frames, crawling tunnels, stools, small tables, play pens, nappy changing tables

Basisgemeinde Wulfshagenerhütten
24214 Gettorf
Tel. 04346/368010
www.basisgemeinde.de
Pikler and Hengstenberg play things

Massivholz-Schreinerei, Gemeinschaft Kehna
Kenenstraße 3,
35096 Kehna
Tel. 06421/974490
email: kehna@t-online.de
www.in-kehna.de
toddler wheel barrows

Intanäschenäl Michael Hühnepohl
Lange Wand 1, 49638 Nortrup
Tel. 05436/902223
www.leiterwagen.de
hand carts from small to large sizes

Stillen, Hüllen, Pflegen Inge Heine
Halberschlaiheide 1,
70794 Filderstadt-Bolanden
Tel. 0711/77036121
email: inge.heine@posteo.de
baby clothes in wool and cotton, soft-felted nappies, thin flannelette towels, thick flannelette towels, flannelette face cloths and much more for the baby

Kinderspielkunst
www.kinderspielkunst.de
climbing tree or an artistically designed climbing frame for outside

Literature

Allwörden, Margret von; **Wiese**, Marie: *Vorbereitete Umgebung für Babys und kleine Kinder. Handbuch für Familien, Krippen und Krabbelstuben (prepared surroundings for infants and toddlers – handbook for families, crèches and toddler groups)*. Pikler Gesellschaft Berlin 2005.

Blechschmidt, Erich: *Der menschliche Embryo (the human embryo)*. 2nd edition Stuttgart 1963.

Blom, Ria; **Charpey**, Thomas; **Barendrecht**, Susanne: *Wenn Babys häufig schreien – Wirksame Hilfe durch Rhythmus und Pucken (when babies cry frequently – effective help using rhythm and swaddling)*. Stuttgart 2005.

Bopp, Annette; **Krohmer**, Birgit: *Der Baby-Guide fürs erste Jahr. Pflege – Entwicklung – Gesundheit – Alltag (Guide to the baby's first year – care, development, health, everyday life)*. München 2010.

Bowlby, John; **Ainsworth**, Mary D. (Ed.): *Deprivation of Maternal Care*. New York 1966.

Bruce, Tina: *Learning Through Play: For Babies, Toddlers and Young Children (Introduction to Child Care)*. London 2011.

Bühler, Walther: *Die meditative Madonnenbildserie (Series of meditative Madonnas)*. Novalis, Nr. 12, 1, 1993/94.

Compani, M.L.; **Lang**, Peter, Ed.: *Waldorfkindergarten heute: Eine Einführung (Waldorf Kindergartens today – an introduction)*. Verlag Freies Geistesleben, Stuttgart 2001.

Czimmek, Anna: Emmi Pikler: *Mehr als eine Kinderärztin (Emma Pikler – more than a children's doctor)*, München.

Delius, Eberhard: *Reismann, Marian, Beziehungen. Fotografien. Mit Bildseiten. Einführung von Anna Tardos*. Pikler Gesellschaft Berlin 1991.

Dornes, Martin: *Der kompetente Säugling. Die präverbale Entwicklung des Menschen (the competetent infant. The pre-verbal development of the human being)*. Frankfurt/M., 14th edition 2009.

Emecheta, Buchi: Gwendolin. In: *Töchter Afrikas (daughters of Africa)*. 2nd edition München 1998.

Fels, Nicola; **Knabe**, Angelika; **Maris**, Bartholomeus: *Ins Leben begleiten. Schwangerschaft und erste Lebensjahre (accompanying the start of life – pregnancy and the first years)*. Stuttgart 2003.

Fernyhough, Charles: *Das Kind im Spiegel (the child in the mirror)*. München 2010.

Fröbel, Friedrich; **Lange**, Wichard: *Gesammelte pädagogische Schriften (collected educational texts)*. Biblio Verlag 1966.

Fuchs, Thomas: *Das Gehirn – ein Beziehungsorgan. Eine phänomenologisch-ökokogische Konzeption (the brain a relationships organ – a phenomenological-ecological concept)*. Stuttgart 2010.

Gebauer, Karl; **Hüther**, Gerald: *Kinder brauchen Wurzeln. Neue Perspektiven für eine gelingende Entwicklung (children need to have roots, new perspectives for a successful development)*. Düsseldorf/Zürich 2005.

Glöckler, Michaela: *Elternsprechstunde. Erziehung aus Verantwortung. Schicksalsfragen – Entwicklungsstufen – Alleinerziehende – Unruhe – Angst – Aggressivität – Behinderungen – Erziehung zur Liebefähigkeit (discussions with parents, ques-

tions of destiny – single parent, discontent, fear, anxiety, aggression, hindrances – educating the capacity to love). Stuttgart 2008 (7th edition 2006).

Glöckler, Michaela; Göbel, Wolfgang: *Kindersprechstunde. Ein medizinisch-pädagogischer Ratgeber. Erkrankungen – Bedingungen gesunder Entwicklung – Erziehungsfragen aus ärztlicher Sicht (consultations about children, a medical-educational guide, illnesses – conditions for healthy development, educational issues from a medical perspective)*. Stuttgart, 18th, re-worked edition. 2010.

Goethe, Johann Wolfgang von: *Warum gabst du uns die tiefen Blicke (why did you cast such a deep gaze on us)*. In: *Sämtliche Gedichte (collected verses)*. Berlin 2007.

Grah-Wittich, Claudia: *Frag nicht – liebe mich einfach (don't ask, just love me)*. In: M.L. Compani, Peter Lang, Ed., *Wie werden aus Jungs richtige Männer? (how can boys become true men?)*. Esslingen 2011.

Grah-Wittich, Claudia: *Pflege der Kindheit als Fundament für Selbstbestimmung und Bindungsfähigkeit (childhood care – fundamental for self-determination and connection)*. In: Andreas Neider (Ed.), *Krisenbewältigung, Widerstandsfähige soziale Bindungen im Kindes- und Jugendalter (mastering crises, resilient social commitments during childhood and youth)*. Stuttgart 2011.

Grah-Wittich, Claudia: *Quasselliese und Zappelphilipp*. In: Andreas Neider (Ed.), *Brauchen Jungen eine andere Erziehung als Mädchen? (do boys need a different education to girls?)*. Stuttgart 2007.

Grah-Wittich, Claudia: *Autonomes Lernen von Anfang an (autonomous learning from the beginning)*. In: Andreas Neider (Ed.), *Autonom lernen – intuitiv verstehen (autonomous learning – intuitive understanding)*. Stuttgart 2008.

Heine, Rolf: *Das Konzept der Zwölf pflegerischen Gesten (the twelve care gestures)*. In: L. de la Houssaye, *Beiträge zur Entwicklung der Anthroposophischen Pflege (contributions towards the development of anthroposophical nursing)*. Dornach 2005.

Heine, Rolf; Bay, Frances (Ed.): *Anthroposophische Pflegepraxis (anthroposophical care in practice)*. Stuttgart, 2nd re-worked and extended edition 2001.

Hüther, Gerald: *Bedienungsanleitung für ein menschliches Gehirn (operating manual for the human brain)*. Göttingen, 2nd edition 2002.

Hüther, Gerald: *Wohin? Wofür? Weshalb? Über die Bedeutung innerer Leitbilder für die Hirnentwicklung (Where to? What for? Why? About the importance of leading inner images for brain development)*. In: Gebauer; Hüther (Ed.), *Kinder suchen Orientierung. Anregungen für eine sinnstiftende Erziehung (children seek orientation – suggestions for a sense-endowed education)*. Düsseldorf/Zürich 2002.

Hüther, Gerald; Krens, Inge: *Das Geheimnis der ersten drei Monate. Unsere frühesten Prägungen (the mystery of the first three months – our earliest influences)*. Düsseldorf, 2nd edition 2003.

Kolzowa, Mariela: *Untersuchungen zur Sprachentwicklung (research into the de-*

velopment of speech). Journal «Der Kinderarzt», 1975/6.

König, Karl: *The First Three Years of the Child – Walking, Speaking, Thinking*. Second revised edition. Floris Books 2004.

Laewen, Hans-Joachim; **Andres**, Beate; **Hedervari**, Eva: *Die ersten Tage – ein Modell zur Eingewöhnung in Krippe und Tagespflege (the first days – a model for acclimatizing to the play group and day care)*. Berlin 2003.

Laewen, Hans-Joachim; **Andres**, Beate; **Hedervari**, Eva: *Ohne Eltern geht es nicht: Die Eingewöhnung von Kindern in Krippe und Tagespflege (without parents it won't work – acclimatizing children to crèche and day care situations)*. Berlin 2006.

Lutzker, Peter: *Der Sprachsinn. Sprachwahrnehmung als Sinnesvorgang (the sense of word, perceiving speech as a sensory process)*. Stuttgart 1996.

Moeller, Michael Lukas: *Die Wahrheit beginnt zu zweit (truth begins together)*. Reinbek bei Hamburg 1995.

Moore, Keith L.: *Embryologie*, 3rd edition Stuttgart 1990.

Neider, Andreas: *Autonom lernen – intuitiv verstehen. Grundlagen kindlicher Entwicklung (autonomous learning – intuitive understanding)*. Stuttgart 2008.

Neider, Andreas: *Krisenbewältigung, Widerstandskräfte, Soziale Bindungen im Kindes- und Jugendalter (mastering crises, resilient social commitments during childhood and youth)*. Stuttgart 2011.

Nuber, Robert R. (Ed.): *Die heilende Madonnenbildreihe nach Felix Peipers und Rudolf Steiner (the healing series of Madonna pictures from Felix Peipers and Rudolf Steiner)*. Stuttgart 1997.

Opp, Günther; **Fingerle**, Michael; **Freytag**, Andreas (Ed.): *Was Kinder stärkt. Erziehung zwischen Risiko und Resilienz (what strengthens children – education between risk and resilience)*. München/Basel 1999.

Patzlaff, Rainer: *Der gefrorene Blick. Physiologische Wirkungen des Fernsehens und die Entwicklung des Kindes (the frozen look. Physiological effect of television and child dvelopment)*. 3rd edition Stuttgart 2004.

Piaget, Jean; **Inhelder**, Bärbel: *Die Psychologie des Kindes (the psychology of the child)*. Olten 1973.

Pikler, Emmi: *Friedliche Babys – zufriedene Mütter. Pädagogische Ratschläge einer Kinderärztin (peaceful babies – content mother. Educational suggestions of a pediatrician)*. Freiburg/Brsg.

Pikler, Emmi: *Laßt mir Zeit! Die selbständige Bewegungsentwicklung des Kindes bis zum freien Gehen. Untersuchungsergebnisse, Aufsätze und Vorträge, aus dem Nachlass zusammengestellt und überarbeitet (give me time – the independent development of a child's movement until it can walk freely. A collection of re-worked lectures and essays from the archive)*. München, 3rd edition 2001 (4th edition 2009).

Pikler, Emmi; **Tardos**, Anna: *Miteinander vertraut werden. Wie wir mit Babys und kleinen Kindern gut umgehen – ein Ratgeber für junge Eltern (learning to trust one another, how to get on well with babies and small children – a guide for young parents). Freiburg/ Brsg., 10th edition 2010.

Pikler, Emmi; **Tardos**, Anna; **Valentin**, Laura; **Valentin**, Lienhard: *Miteinander vertraut werden. Erfahrungen und Gedanken zur Pflege von Säuglingen und Kleinkindern (learning to trust one another, experiences and ideas concerning the care of infants)*. Freiburg/Brsg., 3rd edition 2002 (5th edition 2008).

Reismann, Marian, *Beziehungen. Fotografien. Einführung von Anna Tardos (connections, photographs, introduction by Anna Tardos)*. Ed. Eberhard Delius. Berlin 1991.

Schiller, Friedrich: *Wallensteins Tod III,13 (Wallenstein's death III)*.

Schnabel, Michael: *Die Vielfalt kindlichen Zeiterlebens (the diversity of a child's experience of time)*, liga-kind.de/fk-510-schnabel, 5/10, abgerufen 12.4.2018.

Souci, Fachmann, Kraut: *Die Zusammensetzung der Lebensmittel (the nature of food)*. 7th edition Stuttgart 2008.

Steiner, Rudolf:
The Study of Man. **GA 293**. Rudolf Steiner Press 2004 – lecture 1 and 11.
Anthroposophy as Cosmosophy. **GA 207, GA 208**. Lectures of September, October and November 1921.
Anthroposophy – a Fragment. **GA 45**, concerning hearing and speaking. Dornach 1951.
The Answers of Spiritual Science to the Big Questions of Existence. **GA 60**, Rudolf Steiner Archive 2015 – lecture of 12th January 1911 in Berlin.
The True Nature of the Second Coming. **GA 118**, Rudolf Steiner Press 1971 – lecture of 15th May 1910.
Der Mensch in seinem Zusammenhang mit dem Kosmos – the human being and his connection to the cosmsos. **GA 203**, volume 3, Dornach 1978.
The Renewal of Education. **GA 301**, Anthroposophic Press 2001 – lecture of 10th May 1920 in Basel.
The Education of the Child in the Light of Anthroposophy. **GA 34**, Rudolf Steiner Press 1965.
Occult science, an outline. **GA 13**, Rudolf Steiner Press 1979.
The Spiritual Guidance of the Individual and Humanity. **GA 15**, Anthroposophic Press 1991.
Soul Economy and Waldorf Education. **GA 303**, Anthroposophic Press 1986 – lecture 7.
Die menschliche Seele in ihrem Zusammenhang mit göttlich-geistigen Individualitäten (the human soul and its connection with divine-spiritual individualities). **GA 224** – lectures of 28th and 29th April 1923.
Rosicrucianism Renewed – the Unity of Art, Science and Religion. **GA 284**, Anthroposophic Press 2007 – lecture of 15th October 1911.
The Child's Changing Consciousness and Waldorf Education. **GA 306**, Rudolf Steiner Press 1988 – lecture 6, 20th April 1923.
A Road to Self-Knowledge. **GA 17**. Rudolf Steiner Publishing 1975.
Gebete für Mütter und Kinder (prayers for mothers and children). Dornach 1994.

Curative Education. **GA 317**. Rudolf Steiner Press 1972.

The Education of the Child in the Light of Anthroposophy. **GA 34**. Rudolf Steiner Press 1965.

Metamorphoses of the Soul, Paths of Experience. **GA 59**. Rudolf Steiner Press 1983 – lecture of 14th March 1910.

World History in the Light of Anthroposophy. **GA 233**. Rudolf Steiner Press 1977.

Life between Death and Rebirth. **GA 140**. Anthroposophic Press 1968 – lecture of 11th October 1913.

Meditations for the Time of Day and Seasons of the Year. **GA 267**. Rudolf Steiner Press 2018.

Calendar of the Soul. **GA 40**. Hawthorn Press 1990.

Knowledge of the Higher Worlds and its Attainment. **GA 10**. Anthroposophic Press 1947.

Where and How does One Find the Spirit? **GA 57**. Rudolf Steiner Archive 2015 – lecture of 29th April 1909: *Isis and Madonna*.

Steiner, Rudolf; **Wegman**, Ita: Fundamentals of Therapy. **GA 27**, Chapter 1. Dornach 1925.

Strub, Ute; **Tardos**, Anna (Ed.): *Im Dialog mit dem Säugling und Kleinkind (in conversation with infants and small children)*. Pikler Gesellschaft Berlin 2006.

Vagedes, Jan; **Soldner**, Georg: *Das Kinder-Gesundheitsbuch. Kinderkrankheiten ganzheitlich vorbeugen und heilen (book on child health – preventing and treating illness in a holistic way)*. München 2008.

Vincze, Maria: *Schritte zum selbständigen Essen (steps towards eating independently)*. Pikler Gesellschaft Berlin 1992.

Vincze, Maria: *Mütterliche Liebe – Professionelle Liebe (maternal love, professional love)*. München 2002.

Winnicott, Donald: *Transitional objects and transitional phenomena*. In: International Journal of Psychoanalysis, 1953. 252.

About the authors

Blom, Ria, born 1949. Worked from 1985 in the field of mother and child care as a nurse for children aged 0–4 at the anthroposophical health centre in Utrecht. Since 1994 she has been researching the effects of applying the traditional swaddling technique to restless babies. She is the author of her book «*Wenn Babys häufig schreien: Wirksame Hilfe durch Rhythmus und Pucken*» (Babies that cry frequently – effective help through rhythm and swaddling). www.debakermat.nl.

Compani, Marie-Luise, born 1954 in Darmstadt. Author, co-publisher of «*Waldorfkindergarten heute – Eine Einführung*» (Waldorf Kindergartens today – an introduction). She is a Waldorf educator and teaches on the Waldorf Kindergarten seminar in Stuttgart.

Glöckler, Michaela, Dr. med., born 1946 in Stuttgart. Pediatrician, school doctor and former leader of the Medical section at the Goetheanum (1989–2016). Active lecturing and training doctors at home and abroad. Has produced a number of publications such as: «*Medizin an der Schwelle* (medicine on the threshold)», «*Begabung und Behinderung (gifts and hindrances)*», «*Macht in der zwischenmenschlichen Beziehung* (power in human relationships)», and together with Wolfgang Goebel «*Kindersprechstunde* (child consultations)», «*Spirituelle Ethik* (spiritual ethics)» and others.

Grah-Wittich, Claudia, born 1957, married with 3 children. MA Dipl. in history of art and philosophy. Social worker. Parental advice and child assistance at the institute of «Der Hof» in Niederursel. There she also gives adult education lectures. She is co-responsible for the further training – «Advising parents to see children with new eyes». Gives lectures and seminars at home and abroad. Works with AKK. Various publications.

Heine, Inge, married with three grown up children, nurse and health visitor. Breast feeding and lactation advisor (with IB-CLC). Parental consultant, engaged with the further education and training of women educators. Manager of young child groups (children play – adults learn). Parental guidance in the context of the medical-pedagogical centre at the Filderklinik. Wet nurse.

Heine, Rolf, born 1960, married with 3 children. Nurse and health advisor. Consultant for anthroposophic health care (IFAN). Coordinator of the International Forum for Anthroposophic Nursing. Engaged with training, further training, practical nursing. Publications in books, magazines on the themes of anthroposophical nursing, care of the dying, care of the young child.

Huisinga, Brigitte, born 1949, 3 children, social worker, family counsellor within the context of the young persons welfare office. Family education at «der Hof» in Niederursel since 1984. Between 2002 and 2014 she founded and directed the crèche at «der Hof» in Niederursel. Pikler lecturer.

Jenkinson, Sally. Author of «*Genius of Play: Celebrating the Spirit of Childhood*».

Knabe, Angelika, born 1951, married with 6 children. Founded and developed the Waldorf Kindergarten in Weimar, leading the group there for 15 years. Now manages the Kindergarten. Lecturing and consulting at home and abroad. Member of AKK. Co-author of «*Ins Leben begleiten* (accompanying the start of life)».

Krohmer, Birgit, Freiburg, educator, Waldorf teacher, Pikler lecturer, eurythmy therapist. Co-publisher of «*Der Baby-Guide fürs erste Jahr: Pflege – Entwicklung – Gesundheit – Alltag (Guide to the baby's first year – care, development, health, everyday life)*».

Kühne, Petra, Dr. sc. agr., Frankfurt am Main, married with 3 adult sons. Nutritional scientist, director of the Arbeitskreis für Ernährungsforschung e.V. (nutrition research working group) in Bad Vilbel. Editor of the nutrition journal «*Ernährungsrundbrief*». Contributes to magazines, gives lectures and seminars. Several books: «*Säuglingsernährung* (baby nutrition)» – 10th edition in 2010, co-authored «*Ernährung und Krebs* (nutrition and cancer)» – 6th edition 2006, «*Ernährung und degenerative Erkrankungen* (nutrition and degenerative disease)» (2006), «*Anthroposophische Ernährung – Lebensmittel und ihre Qualität* (anthroposophical nutrition – food and its quality)» (2008), «*Gewürze und Kräuter* (spices and herbs)» (2008).

Looij, Hanne, born 1960 in the Netherlands. Waldorfseminar (Vrije Pedagogische Academie, now called Helicon) in Zeist, history of art at the university of Utrecht. For seven years ran a crèche in Zeist and lectured on education. Founded her own centre in 2005 called Bride, Bureau voor het kleine kind (office for the young child) offering: further training courses, advice to those responsible for young children, courses for parents, talks at parents' evenings.

Mackensen, Ina von, 4 children, Waldorf Kindergarten teacher. Set up and has managed a crèche in the Prenzlauer Berg Waldorf Kindergarten in Berlin since 1997. Family centre, helped develop the further training in infant care and education. Works with AKK and WIFC.

Meinecke, Christoph, Dr. med., Specialist in children and adolescents, psychotherapy. Lead doctor in the field of social pediatrics at the community hospital of Havelhöhe. Works as school doctor in Stuttgart und Berlin. Now works free lance as well as looking after the new born at the community hospital in Havelhöhe. Development of a strategy for early prevention at Havelhöhe through which parents to be can find support and orientation when their children are born. He is manager of the Family Forum in Havelhöhe.

Offenborn, Katharina, born 1959 in Vienna. 3 children. Occupational therapist. Worked for 9 years in the forensic department. Since 2007 has been a free lance lecturer for the Medical Section. Has had a qualified nursing position since 2009. Currently helping to build a crèche in Dinkelscherben near Augsburg.

Winkler, Madeleen, born 1952, GP since 1983 and a doctor at the infant care centre in Gouda, Holland. Published brochures on how to decide on whether to vaccinate and about organ transplants.

Wutte, Elisabeth, Anthroposophical Therapeutic Speech Practitioner.

To the Pictures

All pictures are with the kind permission of the authors: Annette Bopp, Charlotte Fischer, Claudia Grah-Wittich, Brigitte Huisinga, Ina von Mackensen.

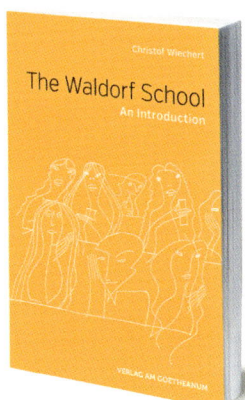

Christof Wiechert
The Waldorf School
An Introduction

120 pages | paperback
ISBN 978-3-7235-1539-6

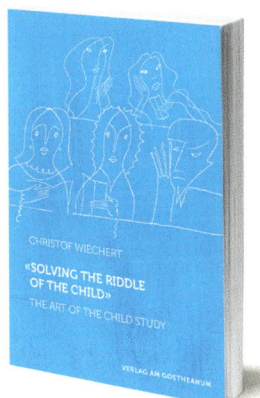

Christof Wiechert
«Solving the Riddle of the Child»
The Art of Child Study

232 pages | paperback
ISBN 978-3-7235-1527-3

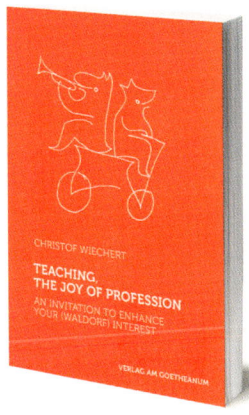

Christof Wiechert
Teaching – The Joy of Profession
An Invitation to Enhance Your (Waldorf) Interest

184 pages | paperback
ISBN 978-3-7235-1473-3

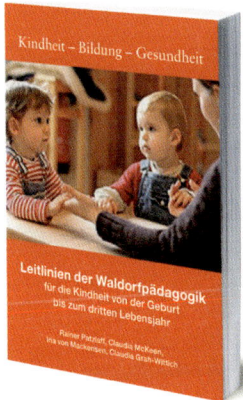

The Guidelines of Waldorf Pedagogy

Edited by the Pedagogical Research Facility at the Bund der Freien Waldorfschulen e.V., Wagenburgstraße 6, 70184 Stuttgart,
im Auftrag der Vereinigung der Waldorfkindergärten e.V. und des Bundes der Freien Waldorfschulen e.V.

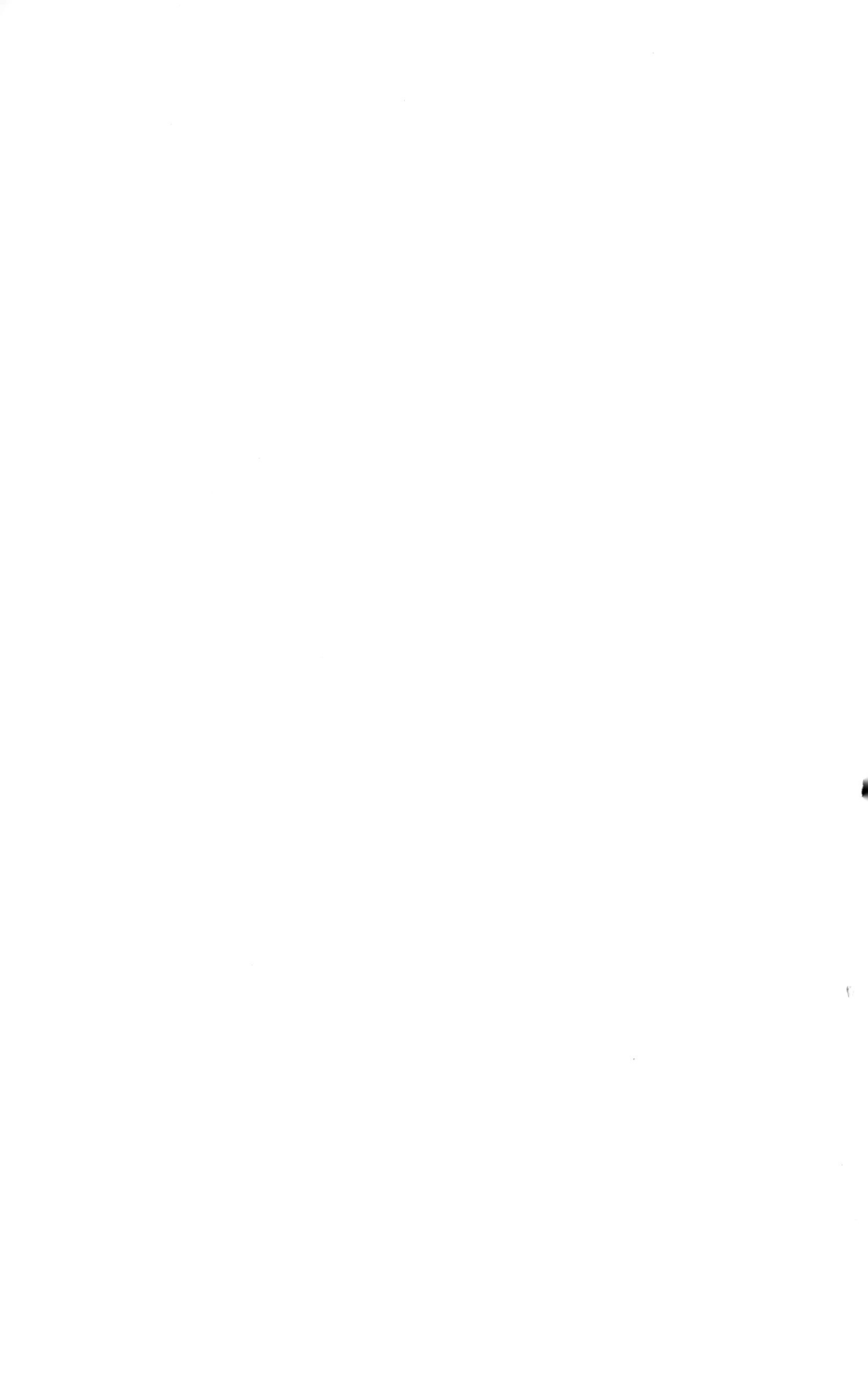